Heal

Eye Problems with Herbs, Minerals and Vitamins

Max Crarer

This book is dedicated to the thousands of health researchers all over the world who are seeking to discover the intricacies of the life of human cells. In particular, the cell's dependence on vitamins, minerals, enzymes, flavonoids, bioflavonoids, etc, to maintain perfect health, the lack of which brings on such eye deficiency troubles as cataracts, glaucoma and macular degeneration, to name but three.

ZEALAND PUBLISHING HOUSE
Private Bag 12029, Tauranga. New Zealand.

First published July 1996 by Max Crarer, Wairoa, New Zealand as "Healing and Reversing Eye and Other Problems With Herbal, Mineral and Vitamin Supplements." (No ISBN number.)
2nd Edition Aug 1997 ISBN 0-908850-21-2
3rd Edition Mar 1999 Revised
Reprinted Nov 1999 Revised
4th Edition Oct 2005 Revised and edited by health researcher David Coory, at request of Max Crarer prior to his death in 2001. Also re-titled as "Heal Your Eye Problems with Herbs, Minerals and Vitamins."
Reprinted July 2007
Reprinted April 2011

Further copies of this book can be obtained by contacting:
Zealand Publishing House Ltd (trading as Health House)
Private Bag 12029, Tauranga, New Zealand.

Phone 0800 140-141 (NZ only) or International +64 3 520-8103
Fax 0800 140-142 (NZ only) or International +64 7 543-0493
Internet www.healthhouse.co.nz

ISBN 0-908850-21-2

Information in this book is not advanced with the intention of curing all eye conditions, but when acted upon in good faith it has been successful in treating many eye conditions considered incurable by most ophthalmologists.

However there is no magic potion. You will not consume one tablet and your eyes will be healed. It will require daily dedication to replace what is lacking in your diet. And when healing occurs, unless you maintain the vitamin and mineral intake to some degree, the condition will return.

Cost may be a factor unable to be overcome by some who barely exist on their present income.

Max Crarer

CONTENTS

Why I wrote this book

Towards the end of 1996, the management of a South Island Hospital, under much criticism from the public (it being election year), decided to import an Australian ophthalmologist to try to reduce the over two year waiting list for operations to remove cataracts.

After advertising for and finding an ophthalmologist to perform their operations, they ran into an unforeseen snag. The NZ Ophthalmologists Union refused to grant the outsider a licence to perform operations in our country.

Why?

Well, a spokesperson explained, the man would be taking money from privately employed NZ ophthalmologists who were quite capable of doing all the necessary operations. And what was more, they would even do some extra operations to reduce the waiting list. But the health authorities must realise, that if they operated and reduced the waiting list to the point where people only needed to wait a few months for a free public hospital operation, then their incomes would suffer considerably. Because if people knew they only had to wait a few months, they would not come to them privately.

Wonder no longer

If any among you have wondered why the New Zealand hospital system, despite the tens of millions of dollars spent on 'revamping', is failing ordinary citizens, especially the elderly, by in some cases allowing 50 year waiting lists (for varicose veins) then wonder no longer.

Unless you have to wait a long time for a public hospital operation, you will not boost the incomes of private practitioners.

"Private enterprise delivers better service?"

Since the 1980's our politicians have actively promoted this new doctrine to the nation.

Along with that hope came legislation to destroy unions. And most unions have been destroyed, or emasculated (not to say that many did not deserve that fate) so wages, without union support for ordinary workers have fallen markedly.

But the South Island hospital example shows that it is only the unions of the lower paid that have been squashed, not the unions of the professionals. Indeed their powers have not even been dented. They will decide who can work in our hospitals.

If their incomes look like decreasing because people being blinded by cataracts are being serviced too quickly by public hospitals, then let them suffer another year or two of blindness. That should loosen their purse strings so that professional unions can maintain their top line incomes.

But things are changing for the better

Most people do not need to pay out $3000 plus for an operation on each eye for cataracts when they can be removed by the same method they arrived.

They came because of lack of minerals and vitamins. They can depart just as quickly when those essentials are supplied to our bodies.

In the USA, an ophthalmologist Dr Price-Todd uses only minerals and vitamins to treat most eye conditions. He claims that if multiple vitamins are taken when early cataracts are first diagnosed, they can be removed in nearly 100% of cases.

Here let me say unequivocally that we do need eye surgeons. They are essential for operations on eyes caused by accidents and other factors, and for people who cannot afford to purchase the essential minerals and vitamins their bodies need.

But the sad fact is, from what I have seen and read, that most ophthalmologists are trying to live in the opulence of the past, and will have to be dragged into the 21st century.

They will need to realise that knowledge of how to deal with deficiency eye ailments, (with the aid of the internet) cannot be suppressed any longer.

Even their own ophthalmological journals throughout the world are reporting that cataracts, retinitis pigmentosa (RP) and macular degeneration can be reversed by the use of mineral and vitamin supplements.

They would far better serve their mostly elderly patients by prescribing such treatments and helping them keep their sight.

Is there a cure for supposedly incurable eye ailments?

I certainly do not say so for all cases, but I do say, because I receive letters from people who have reversed their eye conditions, that herbs, minerals and vitamins can heal eyes.

For how many months or years? Who knows? But I do know of very many people whose eye problems are still improving after two years.

"Do as I say, not as I do"

I am assured of the accuracy of this following report:

A woman patient of an ophthalmologist was told she was developing cataracts. She asked him if herbs or minerals would help. She was told rather scornfully that the only thing they could do was give her expensive urine.

A few months later, another woman who was taking herbal treatment for her eyes, saw this same ophthalmologist in her herb shop, purchasing the identical eye treatment she was on. So she passed on this information to the woman patient he had advised not to take them.

Being a woman who stood no nonsense, she tackled the ophthalmologist face to face about him using these products himself while advising her not to. After a good dressing down he mumbled, "We have to live you know."

Providing the essential nutrients a healthy body needs is a better alternative to a failed operation that still demands payment.

An introduction to glaucoma

Thirty two years ago, on a Sunday afternoon, my mother developed a nagging pain in her eye. She put up with the increasing pain for two days, until she visited an ophthalmologist.

But too late! She had lost the sight in her right eye. The other eye was also under high pressure, which was quickly reduced by the use of chemical drops.

Unknown to her, she had lived with untreated glaucoma for many years, until it eventually claimed her sight in one eye.

A successful operation many years later on the other eye prolonged her vision in that eye until death.

In some ways she was lucky. Some people lose the sight in one eye without any pain whatsoever, and then discover the other eye is also too severely damaged to save.

Is glaucoma hereditary?

Ophthalmologists believe glaucoma is hereditary. They have good reason for this belief because glaucoma does run in families. But while this is true, I also believe (unproven as yet) that it runs in families because Mum prepares the meals (especially in earlier days) and it is quite possible that such meals, because of her inherited tastes and preparation, may be continually deficient in certain essential minerals and vitamins.

If for example a family's favourite meal is fish and chips, that same popular meal, deficient in vitamins and good oils, may carry on through to the next generation.

I develop glaucoma

Being alerted to the hidden danger of glaucoma by our mother, our family all reported for yearly checks of our eyes.

Sure enough, some ten to fifteen years later, all three of her sons, including myself, developed glaucoma.

For the next 12 years, twice a day I placed drugs in my eyes.

A simple explanation of glaucoma

So what is glaucoma, and what are the drops for?

Well, the interior of the eyeball is filled with what in medical terms is called an aqueous solution. In layman's language it is 99% pure water. This water is constantly being manufactured by our blood. In fact we have a permanent spring of water in our eyes.

In normal eyes this water pressurises our eyes to stop them from collapsing inwards. At a certain pressure, this drains away through a tiny drainage hole in the front of the eye. However, as we age and become deficient in minerals and vitamins, these holes can gradually block, thus increasing internal eye pressure.

This internal pressure gradually restricts the entry of blood which feeds the light receptors at the back of the eye, and being starved of nutrients they cannot carry out their purpose.

Pressure can also cause the back of the eye to 'fold' causing some vision loss.

The orthodox medical solution

When they diagnose their patients with glaucoma, ophthalmologists prescribe drugs which expand the drainholes and lower the pressure.

But gradually over time, despite the addition of more powerful and unpleasant drugs, and their more frequent usage, plus the addition of further drugs which slow the manufacture of water, the pressure becomes so high that an operation becomes necessary to manually clear the drainage holes, or blindness will result.

How high can pressures rise before damage occurs?

Research doctors cannot agree on this, but you must recognise that you have not got glaucoma because your internal eye pressure is high. You have got glaucoma when the cells at the back of your eye begin to lose their vision because they are starved of nutrients and the high internal eye pressure begins to distort your eye.

Some people can suffer damage even when pressures are

quite low, while others can go for many years with much higher pressures without damage. But many eyes suffer damage when pressures are over 23 Hg.

Researcher W. Leydhecker suggests that about 20% of the population exceed 21 Hg eye pressure, but only 3% will suffer any vision loss. However, when pressure exceeds 23 Hg, 8% will lose vision.

Both eye and blood pressure can vary

Have you ever read or been told, that some people's blood pressure will give a different reading if taken at different times of the day? Even each arm can give a different reading.

The same thing can apply to eye pressures. A 25 Hg

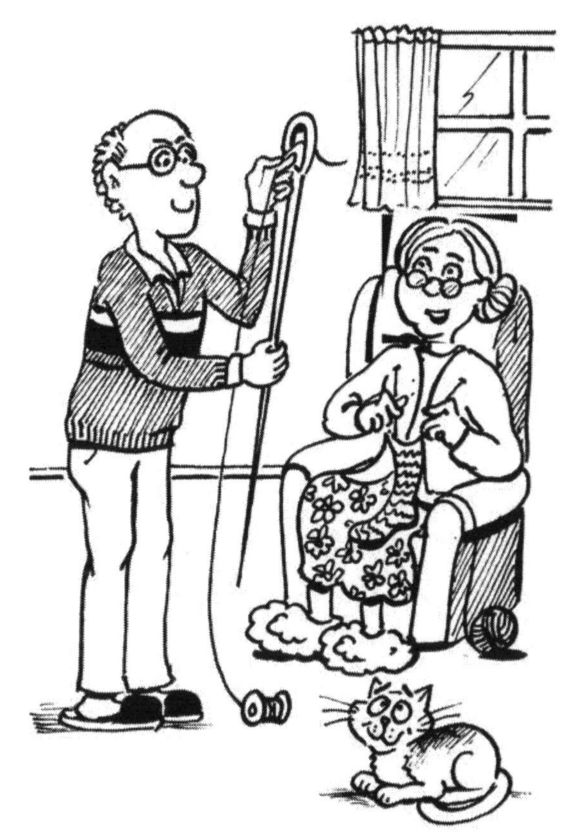

"Yes it will make threading easier dear, but won't it be hell on the clothes?"

reading at ten o'clock in the morning may read only 21 Hg at two o'clock in the afternoon.

How to tell if you have glaucoma

Besides a gradual build up of pressure in the eye, which seldom signifies its presence, a close watch on your peripheral vision can point to eye deterioration.

How can you know for sure if you have glaucoma? You cannot. The only way to find out is to visit an optometrist and have your eyes tested.

A simple cost-free home check

But a cost-free and simple check you can do at home may indicate you have it and that it is affecting your sight. Place your thumbs on the outer edges of your shoulders, (left thumb on left shoulder and right on right) focus your eyes straight ahead and waggle your fingers.

If you cannot detect any finger movement you had better get tested immediately. Glaucoma begins its depredations from the outer edges of your vision.

Usually only one eye affected at a time

I say eye, because it is seldom that both eyes suffer simultaneous damage. But remember this, one person in a hundred will have glaucoma by the age of 40, but ten people in a hundred will have it by the age of 70.

If you are over 40 it is wise to take a glaucoma test from an optometrist.

In New Zealand at present, four people in every hundred have glaucoma. These are official figures, but there are tens of thousands who have never been tested. Some researchers say the incidence could be as high as seven per hundred.

As we continue to live on foods deficient in essential nutrients, the percentage of people with glaucoma in the Western world steadily rises, and will continue to do so.

Researchers claim that by far the best orthodox treatment for glaucoma is a costly operation. However eye surgeons are reluctant to perform this, possibly because of the failure rate (which means blindness), or perhaps if one is cynical, there is the more profitable option of a patient paying a bundle of notes every few months for the rest of their life for a progress report.

How effective is an operation? A friend of mine, operated on one year ago was ecstatic. Sight good, no more drops.

A year later, pressure 27 Hg and rising. Betagan drops again, and the beginnings of cataracts.

How effective are glaucoma eye drops and how safe are they?

Two well known eye researchers, Caputo and Katz have this to say, *'It is sometimes difficult to determine whether treatments are more detrimental than the disease itself.'*

Well, there is considerable evidence that Beta Blocker Drops, which also contain a harmful preservative Benzalkonium Chloride, may actually worsen glaucoma.

While most manufacturers keep silent, one does list the following side effects that can occur in up to one in four patients – Transient eye irritation, eye redness, burning, tearing, swelling, blurred or cloudy vision.

The brand names of these drops are: Timoptic, Betoptic, Ocupress, Betagan and Optiprandol.

Also drops containing Carbonic Anhydrase can cause lethargy, weight loss, fatigue, anorexia and depression.

A survey of glaucoma patients using drops revealed up to 30% experienced side effects, including – congestive heart failure, dizziness, and wheezing.

Are there different types of Glaucoma?

Yes, there are four types.

Angle Closure Glaucoma Specialists say it can only be treated by surgery. They tell us that about cataracts too.

Pigmentary Glaucoma This is a variant of Angle Closure Glaucoma. It has not been known to respond to any degree with nutritional supplements, although herbs and enzymes have yet to be trialled.

Low Tension Glaucoma The latest research suggests the prime cause of low tension Glaucoma is Subclinical Hypothyroidism. Many people unknowingly suffer from this problem and should ask their doctor to test them.

Solely by taking thyroid tablets the response has been less visual loss and improved sight.

Open Angle Glaucoma This appears to have a good response to minerals, vitamins and herbs. Again check that thyroid. Try the Iodine check on page 83.

Can anything be done to ward off Glaucoma?

Yes. Almost all people with glaucoma suffer from a deficiency of Vitamin A and Vitamin D.

All of these are also helpful:

Selenium, Magnesium aspartate, Zinc, Manganese, B vitamins, Iodine, CoQ10.

And the herbs, Ginkgo Biloba, Bilberry, Garlic and Eyebright.

Some of these contain anti-oxidants and bioflavonoids which also help to clear drainage tubes.

If I am diagnosed with glaucoma will eyedrops help?

Will they cure you? No, but in some cases they may delay eye damage for a number of years.

But I believe that the best and safest way to preserve your eyes is to supply your body the necessary nutrients to protect them naturally.

Is glaucoma inevitable as we age?

Yes, increasingly so in the western world. For we consume foodstuffs lacking in essential minerals.

But some people living in mineral-rich areas of the world, with an average age of over a hundred, have never heard of glaucoma.

This would seem to prove that most eye troubles are not diseases caused by bacteria or viruses, but nutritional deficiency problems and can be prevented or reversed with adequate mineral and vitamin intake.

What is the success rate using minerals, vitamins and herbs?

Well it varies from person to person, but in general, if a

person has just been diagnosed, and they are on no other medications, the percentage who receive benefit by way of a pressure drop and better health would be over 90%.

The trouble is, as we age most of us become deficient in many minerals. That deficiency shows up in gall stones, heart troubles or arthritis. Our doctors then put us on three or four different drugs. Some of these act against one another, and most of them destroy vitamins and leach essential minerals from the body.

The remarkable thing is, even some of these people show eye improvement on mineral and vitamin supplement.

A stitch in time saves nine

Prevention is always better than cure. There is evidence to suggest that eye problems and other aliments that show up in our 60's may have their foundation ten years or so earlier. It is only when our bodies have used up all alternatives that deficiency ailments rapidly appear.

Therefore it would be better to take minerals and vitamins from age 40, rather than wait until deficiency ailments appear in our 50's and 60's.

This may be the reason why saturation dosing is sometimes needed to effect a cure.

Monitor your eyes

By checking your vision every six months or so on the black and white squares on page 26 you will not need an ophthalmologist to tell you that you are developing macular failure.

You do not need to pay someone to tell you that you are developing cataracts when your vision begins to become cloudy.

But glaucoma is different. The only person who can tell you if you are coming to this ailment is an ophthalmologist or an optometrist. That is why it is prudent to have your eyes checked for glaucoma once you have hit 40 years of age. What you do if diagnosed adversely then becomes your choice.

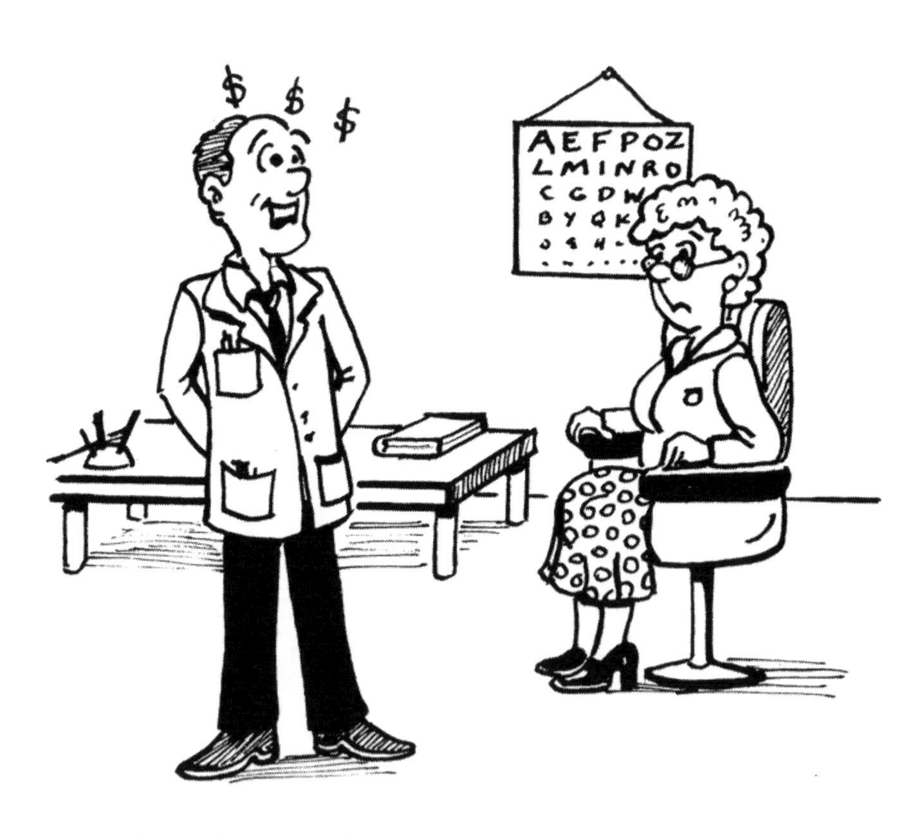

"You have nothing to worry about Mrs Moneybags. It will give me much pleasure to relieve you of your casharacts – er.. sorry... I mean cataracts."

This all started when I healed my own glaucoma

My eyes suddenly test normal

On the morning of the 18th July 1994, I set out on the two hour journey from Wairoa to Hastings for my annual visit to my ophthalmologist. Half way there I remembered I had not put any drops in my eyes that morning.

I reported this fact to my eye specialist as he began his examination. His response was, "That is good. We will get a good test."

An unexpected result

A few minutes later he said "Look, I don't think you need to put any more drops in your eyes. Your pressures are normal."

He told me to return again in one month and he would check me again free of charge.

After receiving assurance that no harm could come to my eyes by not using the eyedrops for a month, I departed.

Another check

Two months later I was re-examined and my pressures were still normal.

Over those two months I had pondered the reasons as to why glaucoma, that had been with me for 12 years should suddenly decide to depart. I formed the opinion that the element Selenium, which I had recently been taking, was responsible.

I asked the specialist if I could look through my records from the time I was first diagnosed as having glaucoma. This we did and found that I had begun using drops some 12 years ago, when the pressure was found to be 25 mm Hg.

Always ask, "What is my pressure?"

Incidentally, in all those years I had never asked what glaucoma was, or what my pressures were. To me glaucoma was like a wart. I had it. It didn't hurt. It was a nuisance.

Provided I put drops in my eyes morning and night every day, all would be well.

Each year the ophthalmologist would say everything is OK and off I would go to carry on with life.

But this time I asked "What is normal pressure?"

I was told anywhere between 14 to 20 Hg.

I told the specialist I thought possibly Selenium had something to do with my eye pressure improvement, as I had been taking Selenium.

His only comment was, "They say Selenium delays the aging process."

Back home I again pondered what had caused my eyes to become normal. What had I been doing to have caused the change?

Searching for reasons

Some two years earlier, a sharp pain in my knee had caused me to visit my doctor. He diagnosed arthritis, but offered no solution.

I remembered that I had read somewhere that many areas of New Zealand were deficient in Selenium, and that it was important to good health. So I began taking 50 micrograms of Selenium a day.

Within two days the pain had gone. I noticed on my records that my eye pressures had begun to return to normal around the same time. So I assumed that it was this trace mineral Selenium that had been the catalyst in removing my high eye pressures.

A good luck call

A month or so later, early one morning I was listening to Radio Pacific when the host asked anyone who had some good luck recently to phone in.

So I rang the host explaining how I had cured my glaucoma by using Selenium.

People from all over New Zealand began phoning me asking how much Selenium was needed to 'cure' their glaucoma.

I decided to keep records of many of them. Alas, a picture soon emerged. Two or three had improvement in sight. Some had reduced pressures. There was one whose cataracts had improved, but for about 95% there was no improvement.

More light from a New Zealand book

Around this time a friend loaned me a book written by New Zealand author David Coory, entitled 'Stay Healthy By Supplying What's Lacking In Your Diet'.

It explained all about minerals and vitamins and the part they played in maintaining a healthy body and showed the foods we need to eat to obtain them. It also listed the health problems that occur when our bodies become deficient in them, or overdose on them.

While reading his book, I discovered that Zinc and the vitamins A, C, and E, were essential for healthy eyes. I recalled that I had been taking Zinc and Vitamin C at various times, months before I began using Selenium.

I presumed then that Selenium was probably essential, but probably only as a catalyst. Everything I have since read about Selenium shows it is essential for healthy muscles. No doubt there are lots of muscles in the eyes, and I have since discovered that it appears to be essential for efficient capillary action in the eyes.

So I told all who contacted me after that to use vitamins A, C, E and Selenium and Zinc.

But alas, even that combination, while helping considerably more people, was not the answer.

An alternative answer

A few months after I first contacted Radio Pacific, I received a circular from Doreen Fisher of Whangarei, a Herbalist and Naturopath.

She said that she sold, among other things, herbal products that were effective in helping many eye conditions.

A little later I received a call from a man named Eric, seeking help with his cataracts. I told him of my own experience with minerals and vitamins, and also of Doreen Fisher whom he knew.

Eric was a keen gardener who did not feel he was in need of minerals and vitamins, so he decided to try the herbal remedy that Doreen suggested.

Three months later his cataracts had disappeared.

A month or two later I received a phone call from Bill, an optometrist in Whangarei. He had recently paid $2000 for an operation on one eye to relieve pressure, and now his ophthalmologist wanted to do the other eye, as the pressure was too high. He asked me for any possible help.

I told him what I knew about minerals and vitamins and suggested that he contact Doreen about herbs, which he did.

Supplements – the new approach

Some weeks later Bill the optometrist phoned me again. After using minerals, vitamins and herbs, his eye pressure had come down 10 points and returned to normal. An operation was no longer necessary.

He had also used a new product Doreen suggested called Pycnogenol with Protectors, one of the world's most powerful anti-oxidants, which also has the ability to help blood flow through the tiniest capillaries.

Because of his own successful treatment, Bill, much to the chagrin of other ophthalmologists in the region began advising people to use supplements, rather than drugs.

I originally thought this combination treatment of herbs, minerals and vitamins was a world breakthrough, but I have since discovered that one or two ophthalmologists throughout the world have been treating their patients with nothing else but supplements for some years.

In fact I have since read in two ophthalmology journals, of two trials using minerals and vitamins, lasting many years, that gave impressive results with macular degeneration, which ophthalmologists still say is untreatable.

One can only marvel that such information has not filtered down to other ophthalmologists.

Treating glaucoma with supplements

Know what your eye pressure is

If you decide to use supplements the first step is to know your eye pressure. So whenever you have your eyes tested, always ask what the pressure is.

The next move is to learn by how much eye drops, if you have been using them, are lowering your pressure.

So stop using the drops for one day and then go to an optometrist and ask for a pressure reading for glaucoma.

You may have to phone around for prices first, because the actual pressure test only takes about two minutes, but some optometrists will want you to do a full eye test for $80 or $60. So shop around in the Yellow Pages. You do not want to be robbed. You only want to pay for the service you ask for. A reasonable price would be $25.

Begin taking supplements then check your pressure again in three weeks time

Having established your pressure, then begin taking your minerals, and vitamins, etc.

After three weeks, return for another check.

If your pressures are on the way down, you are on the right track. If not, try increasing your dosage slightly. Most people, using the right dosage can reduce their pressures by up to 10 points within two months.

If your pressures are moving down, then whether or not you continue to use drops is up to you. You have read in earlier pages what some researchers have to say about their efficiency or otherwise.

How much easier it would be if we could find ophthalmologists who would tolerate natural treatments and monitor our progress.

Could it be that they see natural healing as a threat to their opulent incomes, or is it that their dogmatism has blinded them to the fact that there may be more natural treatments?

Are supplements easier than drops?

In plain language, no. If it were just a matter of placing drops in your eyes once or twice a day and that would keep your sight intact for life, then I would choose drops. But as some researchers tell us, drops in some cases actually worsen the problem of failing eyesight.

So I choose the somewhat harder regime, and it can be a regime. Like drops, you will twice, or even three times a day take tablets instead.

You will need to purchase those supplies and it will cost you a lot more than it costs you for eye drops. However, in favour of this, you will not only be treating your eyes but your whole body. And a day or two without supplements will do you no harm.

How much should I take?

It is impossible to say with certainty that you need this or that. Everybody will be deficient in some things and not others.

It depends on what you eat, or more correctly, what you don't eat. For example, if you eat broccoli leaves, pumpkin, kumara or carrots daily, you would not need any Vitamin A.

You begin to overdose on pre-formed Vitamin A (retinol) at over 1500 micrograms daily. This can produce blurred vision, and in severe cases, peeling skin.

But you cannot overdose on pumpkins, kumara or carrots, which contain the beta carotene form of Vitamin A , or the raw material from which our liver makes Vitamin A. Although too much beta carotene food can produce a yellow tinge to skin, especially the palms.

So the safest way to obtain Vitamin A is from beta carotene in vegetables or beta carotene tablets. Take plenty of it.

Too little Vitamin A puts you up for cataracts, irritable eyes (they feel as if they have grit in them), reduced night vision, and in severe deficiency cases, blindness.

How can I cut down on the amount of supplements I need to take?

You can get hold of a book written by New Zealand

author, David Coory entitled 'Stay Healthy By Supplying What's Lacking In Your Diet'. This book lists all the minerals and vitamins you need and has charts showing which foods to eat to supply all your daily needs.

You will still need to buy some supplements as today's foods are woefully low in minerals.

David's book does not cover herbs, but research scientists around the world are belatedly recognising the remarkable effectiveness of herbs and herbal remedies.

An analysis of most herbs connected with eyes shows that besides alkaloids and enzymes they contain traces of some 25 to 30 minerals, which no doubt provides some reason for their healing properties.

You will need to purchase some herbs to make EW eyewash which I talk about below.

Correct balance important

It is important to remember that it is not only a lack of minerals and vitamins that affect your eyes, but also an imbalance of these, which can cause them to react with one another.

A shortage of Copper for example makes for weak blood vessels, cells and lack of energy, while too much Copper, which is a factor in high blood pressure and arthritis, can only be controlled and removed by adequate levels of Vitamin C and Zinc.

If your doctor is not aware of these imbalances, and takes no tests for them first, you may well end up taking drugs you do not need. True, they may suppress the complaint, but they will not cure it and could well lead to sight damage.

What will it cost me to use supplements?

Well, the sad fact is, plenty. An ophthalmologist can prescribe expensive drugs for our eyes that may be far less effective than what is written here, and in most cases the taxpayer will subsidise the cost.

But even if you find a friendly ophthalmologist, I doubt if the Department of Health would allow prescriptions containing anti-oxidants, minerals, or vitamins. And if you haven't the money to purchase what you need to prevent blindness, well who cares? Least of all politicians who each year cut down pensions for the elderly to below sustenance level but raise their own pay.

To those of you who can afford it, what price can you put on keeping your sight?

The quantities suggested are for a person of say 75 kgs. A person half that weight would take half the amount. To an extent you must use your own discretion. A feed of oysters and you would not need Zinc next day. A day on fruit or fruit juices and you would not need any Vitamin C.

A person on a very balanced nutritional diet may not need the quantities mentioned.

Preparing EW (herbal eye wash)

EW is a traditional herbal eye wash made from golden seal root, bayberry root bark, eyebright herb and red raspberry leaves.

It can also be used internally if so desired. However a new herbal product called Perfect Eyes supersedes this product for internal use.

EW is essential to bathe your eyes if you have cataracts or glaucoma. So here is how to prepare and use it.

I must stress that it is of prime importance to adopt strict hygiene when preparing and using EW. Be sure your eyebath and the glass jar you keep your eyewash in is spotlessly clean.

You will need two glass jars with screw on lids that hold over a cup of water each. The reason for two jars is that when you finish one, you will have time to refill it without haste, as you use the second jar.

Fill them both with distilled water. You can buy distilled water at the supermarket or Warehouse for under $1 a litre. I have tried collecting rainwater but tests have shown it is a long way from being pure.

Also from a supermarket, purchase a packet of coffee filters. These are on the shelf with the coffees. Be sure they are paper ones. These are used to filter your EW solution.

Now take a clean, empty cup and fill it with distilled water, then pour this cup of water into a stainless steel pot and bring to the boil.

Next take a pack of EW capsules and remove two capsules. Twist these two capsules apart and empty the contents into the cup. Squeeze them to make sure all the powder comes out of the capsule.

Now take your boiling water and pour it over the powder in the cup. Leave for 10 minutes or more.

Then take one of your two jars and place two filter papers over the mouth. Pour the EW liquid carefully into the filters. Once you see sediment coming, stop and discard the remaining sediment-laden water.

Filter throughly

The reason I say use two filter papers is that the sediment is extremely fine, and I have found using one filter is not enough to stop some sediment getting through. Even though it is fine, it will still feel like grit if you get it in your eyes.

You will find it takes a long time to filter completely. I hurry the process by lifting the filters, twisting the top, then gently squeezing them.

Pour the filtered EW into your glass jar, and when cold, screw on the top and store it in the refrigerator.

Only use this preparation for 5 days, and then discard it. When it is getting low or old, make another fresh batch in your second jar.

To bathe your eyes

Three quarters fill an eyebath with the eyewash. Lower your head, fit the eyebath into your eye socket, raise your head, open your eye and blink them in the liquid 10 to 20 times. Repeat the procedure with the other eye.

It may sting a little at first, but you will get used to it. It is a good idea to hold a cloth under your eye to stop any drops spilling onto your clothing for they will stain.

If after a few months, when your eyes have become well adjusted to the drops, and you may not have achieved the desired effect, the addition of a tiny pinch of cayenne pepper in the powder will give a much stronger mix. It will sting a little. But be careful, just the tiniest of pinches. Too much pepper will sting strongly and cause your eye to become bloodshot.

In the first few weeks some people may notice a mucous discharge from their eyes, especially when waking. Do not be alarmed, the condition will soon disappear.

A link between caffeine and glaucoma?

Recently I had a letter from a man who reduced his eye pressures from 27 to 15 by doing nothing else but giving up caffeine (no tea, coffee or chocolate).

I imagine for some that would be very hard. But old information I have just read does suggest there is a link between caffeine and glaucoma.

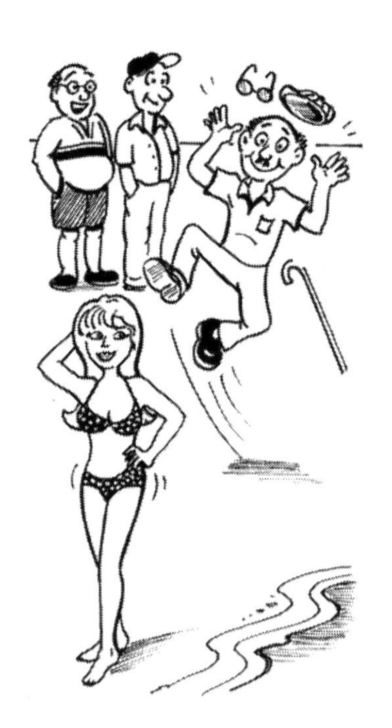

"Must be a miracle! A minute ago Fred's half blind, now he can see."

Macular Degeneration

What is the macula of the eye?

The macula is centred in the retina at the back of the eye. It comprises a circular area about the diameter of a pencil rubber. It contains tens of millions of 'rods' (night vision cells) and 'cones' (day vision cells).

These cells are covered by another layer of some 40,000 cells called the retinal pigment epithelium. Perhaps we could call these cells 'cleaners' because they mop up all the used debris and pass it out into the bloodstream for disposal.

However if these cells become clogged with rubbish, fresh nutrients from the blood cannot enter and the eye is in trouble.

Macular Degeneration is a condition that develops, especially in the aged, when restricted access of blood to the eye (and often other key areas of the body) starves the macula of essential nutrients and elements.

What is the effect of Macular Degeneration?

Macular Degeneration, also known as MD is the exact opposite of Glaucoma. In this case it is the centre of the eye that loses vision.

Sufferers develop a black spot in the centre of the eye (see cover photo) which gradually expands.

Since it is only the centre cells of the eye that record colour, as these cells die the sufferer also gradually loses colour vision and is only able to see in shades of grey.

Orthodox medicine offers no hope to sufferers of Macular Degeneration.

Who is likely to have Macular Degeneration?

Some researchers say that the seeds of Macular Degeneration begins from the age of 30 years.

1% of the population will develop MD by the age of 60.

12% of people aged 65-75 will have it.

27% of people aged 75-85 will have it.

Blue eyed people are more susceptible to MD than others.

There are four factors that clog cells in the macula.

Very high estrogen levels.
High blood sugar levels.
Prolonged stress.
Lack of Vitamin C and other bioflavonoids.

Macular Degeneration generally appears first in only one eye, and may take four years before it appears in the other eye. It does not affect total vision. Your side vision is not impaired, but you will have a black hole in your central vision.

How to test for Macular Degeneration

Once Macular Degeneration has been discovered, the loss of vision progresses slowly.

The first indication that you have it is when a straight line becomes blurred.

You can test yourself on the Grid Pattern below. Always close one eye when doing this as you may not discover it in one eye with both eyes open.

If the centre lines are in any way bent or blurred, it is time to act if you wish to save your sight. But don't run to orthodox 'experts.' All they can do is tell you what you already know and relieve you of a bundle of bank notes.

Macular Degeneration can also be detected during an examination by an ophthalmologist before you become aware of it, because the narrowing of the veins in the eye will be noticed.

Test your eyes for macular trouble on this grid

If the centre lines are in any way bent or blurred, it is time to act if you wish to save your sight.

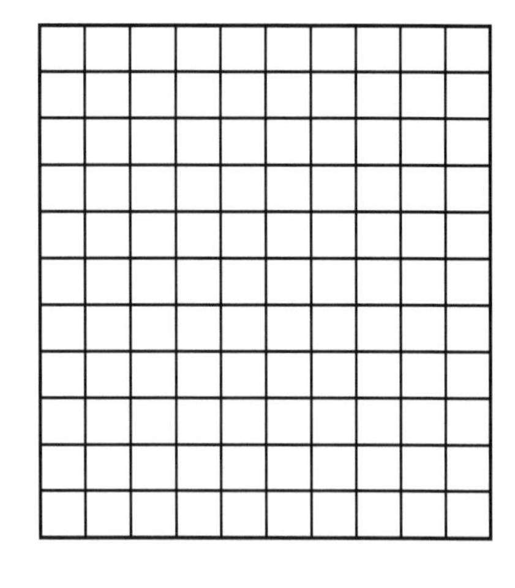

An increase in astigmatism can be an indication of Macular Degeneration?

Astigmatism occurs when the retina of the eye, or sometimes the lens, is slightly distorted and does not focus an image clearly on all planes.

The result is that a person sees partly clearly and partly blurred. It affects about a third of the population, but is usually so slight as to be unnoticeable. A good pair of glasses will easily correct astigmatism.

However many researchers say that an increase in astigmatism is a pointer to oncoming Macular Degeneration.

What is Wet Macular?

Although both have the same cause, there are what is called 'Wet' and 'Dry' Macular Degeneration.

Wet Macular is caused by a rapid deterioration of 'Dry' Macular Degeneration. It is a less common condition, signified by internal bleeding. This occurs when the restricted blood vessels in the retina slowly rupture. This can show as black spots, or as a bigger bleed which will quickly close down your macular vision.

About 10% of Macular Degeneration sufferers progress to 'Wet' Macular.

Often the cause is aspirin or Warfarin (a blood thinner). This is not to be unexpected, as both aspirin, Warfarin and smoking all destroy Vitamin C which is essential for eye health.

Orthodox medicine offers no hope but to seal the bleeding with laser treatment. But sight becomes progressively dimmer.

However Wet Macular also responds to natural remedies.

What can be done to stop or reverse Macular Degeneration?

If you have the money, there are many things that can be done, and tens of thousands of people throughout the world are doing it.

As I have stated elsewhere; Do not regard your

ophthalmologist as a god, and do not believe it if he tells you, "nothing can be done."

Do other people in the world treat eyes as you suggest?

Here is what American ophthalmologist Dr Gary Price-Todd, whose first preference is always to treat eye troubles with vitamins and minerals, has to say about Macular Degeneration.

"In my practice, I find the majority of my patients with Macular Degeneration also have sub-clinical hypothyroidism. These patients respond very favourably to thyroid supplementation. In addition, anti-oxidants, vitamins and minerals favourably affect the course of this disease, improving vision in 88% of my patients."

Miracles can happen

One morning in December 1997, Mr Eckard Onken, 5 Voysey Close, Quakers Hill, 2763, Australia, who is technically blind, phoned me and asked if anything could be done for him.

I suggested he try a combination of minerals, vitamins and herbs.

He also said that his mother was seeing black spots before her eyes and asked if anything could be done for her.

On the 2nd of March, 1998 I received the following fax:

Dear Mr Crarer

Third month into your therapy. My mother 91, dancing black spots have disappeared out of perceived picture.

I 61, can again see the floor is brown, the walls are pink, and the ceilings white. Before 1987 there was only dark and light.

Have patience

I have known and read of people who persevered with minerals, vitamins and herbal treatments for 10 months before improvement was noted. Dr Gary Price-Todd states that in advanced cases, Macular Degeneration improvement may not show up until a year has gone by.

The remarkable thing is however, that once a nourishing

blood supply is restored to the retina, the cells in the macula actually regenerate.

More information

Here is an item gleaned from the Journal of the American Medical Association, volume 272, page 1413, 1994.

"One can only marvel at the ignorance, or inability of ophthalmologists to follow research, when they tell patients there is no cure for macular troubles."

In a study lasting seven years of 100 people on a nutrient diet, including daily, 500 mg of Vitamin C ascorbate, 5400 iu of beta carotene Vitamin A, and 250 mcg of Selenium (this from a nation that supposedly has plenty of Selenium in its food), and 250 mg of Vitamin E.

The result – deterioration of the macula either stopped or improved with 60 people. So do not give up hope.

But I wonder how greater a percentage would have been healed had they also been taking Pycnogenal, B vitamins, Bilberry, Eyebright, Taurine and Ginkgo Biloba?

All these are very beneficial for all eye conditions.

Bilberry for bright light discomfort

If you cannot stand bright light, or find difficulty in dim light, take Bilberry. This herb is excellent for many eye conditions, including sometimes, correcting near sightedness.

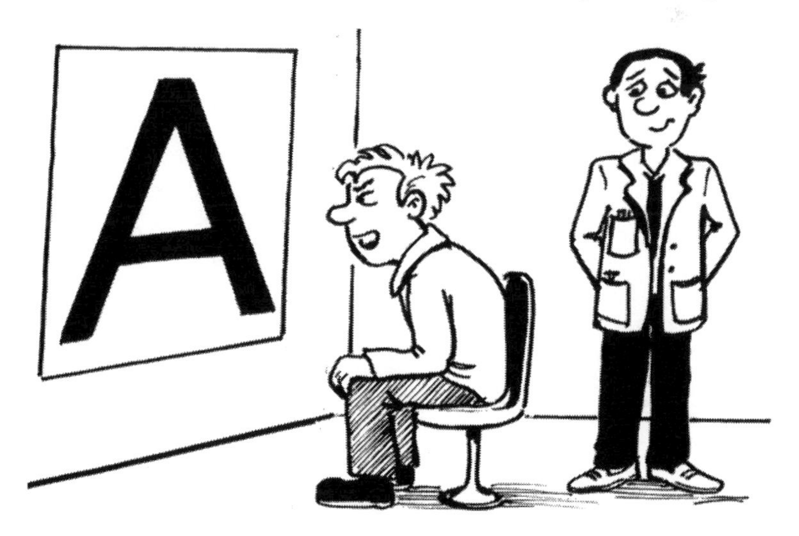

"I can't quite make out the bottom line."

Cataracts

What are cataracts?

Cataracts are an eye condition where the lens of the eye, which is normally crystal clear, becomes cloudy. This leads to increasingly blurred vision. Eventually no light can enter the eye.

It is a condition that usually develops slowly and is seldom seen in people under 50 years of age.

In almost all cases, cataracts are caused by a lack of minerals and vitamins, especially Vitamin A and C, although in some cases a faulty thyroid gland, a diabetic condition, or steroid drugs can be at fault.

Can cataracts be eliminated?

Yes, if remedial action is taken as soon as cataracts are discovered, they can in almost 100% of cases be eliminated. This requires a correct intake of minerals, vitamins and anti-oxidants.

Current treatment of cataracts is to operate and insert a plastic lens (at a price exceeding $3000 in NZ) into the lens sheath.

In most cases this succeeds, but the complication or failure rate, which I believe is about 6%, still requires your cash payment in full.

Supplements on the other hand, enable your eyes to heal naturally. The lens begins to clear from the outer edges and the full clearance generally takes about six months.

And you don't need to visit a specialist to know what's happening, you can tell by your improved sight.

Are there different types of cataracts?

Indeed, there are seven main recognisable types:

Posterior sub-capsular cataracts. In this type the eye finds it very hard to operate in bright lights. This normally signifies a lack of Vitamin A. People who use steroids, or are diabetic, or lack chromium (which is a common factor in diabetics), or have a thyroid deficiency are the ones who are more prone to develop this type of cataract.

Minimum treatment for this type of cataract is to take daily as follows:

75,000 iu	Vitamin A in the form of beta carotene.
400 mcg	Chromium GTF (glucose tolerance factor).
1000 mg	Vitamin C.
4	Multi-vitamin tablets.*
200 mg	Pycnogenol (anti-oxidant).

In addition check for thyroid malfunction, and stop taking steroids.

Opalescent cataracts. People who have trouble with milk products are prone to this type, as are diabetics. Easily reversed if you take daily:

25,000 iu	Vitamin A as beta carotene.
1000 mg	Vitamin C.
4	Multi-vitamin tablets.*

Brunescent cataracts. In this type, melanin, produced in the eye, colours the lens brown. The fact that this protective colouring is occurring would suggest the eye is being exposed to strong sunlight, or perhaps arc welding glare. It also suggests a lack of anti-oxidants in the blood.

Suggested treatment: Wear sunglasses that filter out ultra-violet light, and take daily:

1500 mg	Vitamin C.
200 mcg	Selenium.
250 mg	Glutathione (amino acid anti-oxidant).
200 mg	Vitamin E.
4	Multi-vitamin tablets.*
200 mg	Pycnogenol.
600 mg	Omega 3 flax oil capsules.

Cortical Spoking and Water Clefts cataracts. These are nutritional deficiency cataracts. Suggested treatment is to take daily:

10,000 iu	Vitamin A as beta carotene.
4 tablets	Pycnogenol.
4	Multi-vitamin tablets.*

Nuclear Sclerosis cataracts. This type of cataract is always identified by deficiencies in the diet associated with the aging process. Suggest treatment is to take daily:

200 mcg	Selenium.
200 mg	Vitamin E.
100,000 iu	Vitamin A as beta carotene.
200 mg	Pycnogenol.
1000 mg	Vitamin C.
4	Multi-vitamin tablets.*
250 mg	Glutathione (amino acid anti-oxidant).
1000 mg	Omega 3 fish oil.

* **Note:** In all cases above, where 4 Multi-vitamin tablets are suggested, reduce that to 2 tablets after four weeks.

Ask "What type of cataract is it?"

So if your ophthalmologist tells you that you have a cataract forming, ask 'What type of cataract is it?'

If he or she doesn't know, then you can be sure they are not up with the play regarding cataracts.

Also bear this in mind, the professional dealing with you relies on you for their income. You have a right to know.

Wear a hat

It was once believed that exposure to the sun over a long period of time could cause a protein build-up in the eye, leading to cataracts. Perhaps there is still some validity in that. But modern researchers now believe that lack of the vitamins A, C, and E, and lack of the minerals Zinc and Selenium are the prime cause of cataracts.

It is worth recalling that the body cannot uptake Zinc or Iron unless it has adequate levels of Vitamin B6 (pyridoxine). Some other B vitamins are also essential for eye health.

But wear a hat in the summer sun anyway. Exposure to too much ultraviolet light can cause problems, and not only to your eyes.

Ultra-violet light damage to old eyes

Over age 50, when we begin to lose the ability to diligently process all anti-oxidants from our foods, our eyes become more vulnerable to the constant hail of photons from light on the retina of our eyes.

The enemy that does the most damage is ultra-violet light. These light particles drive deep into our eyes whenever direct sunlight strikes them.

Just as a spoon held over a candle gathers particles of soot, so the eyes of people exposed to sunlight gather debris from damage by light. These garbage deposits occur in all eyes that are not totally guarded by blood saturated with anti-oxidants. They form damage spots on the retina called drusen.

Blue eyed blondes beware

Constant bombardment of the retina, especially for people with blue eyes, who are more susceptible to sunlight damage, eventually weakens the retina and macular degeneration sets in.

It is important for people in New Zealand, and absolutely essential for any person with serious eye trouble, to wear wrap-around sunglasses that filter out ultra-violet light.

Beware of phoney ultra-violet sunglasses

If you are buying a pair of wrap around sunglasses, be sure to take them outside and look through them at the blue sky. It should look grey.

If the sky does not look grey, you can be certain that the glasses you have are not filtering ultra-violet light. Watch for this. Some manufactures are not honest.

A good pair of ultra-violet filtering glasses would seldom be purchased at under $200 in New Zealand. You can buy such glasses in America for NZ$160, so don't be robbed in New Zealand by paying $400 for them.

Any person who comes in from working in the garden and has difficulty adjusting to the shade, is a candidate for macular trouble.

"I'm okay, I've had my cataracts removed"

No! No! No! You more than anyone need sunglasses.

If you have had cataract surgery, sunglasses are doubly important. What most people who have had surgery do not realise, and are never told by their ophthalmologists (perhaps they don't know themselves), is that once the sliver of skin on the original lens is removed, it exposes the retina to direct, unfiltered sunlight. When this occurs the retina can be damaged six times faster than normal.

Cataracts are caused by protein build-up in the lens of the eye. It may actually be nature's protection against light damage to the retina. Outdoor people who work in direct sunlight are far more prone to cataracts than others.

The facts are, that the protein build-up in the lens has occurred because of a lack of anti-oxidants to protect the eye. Many people are surprised to find that within a year in some cases, that defence mechanism has again caused the skin of the lens sheath (which holds the new plastic lens in place) to cloud over, and again their vision has become blurred.

One way to keep a young eye for old age

When surgeons removed a dense cataract from an 80 year old man, they found an eye whose retina appeared 30 years younger than normal.

Naturally healed cataracts can return

Cataracts cause up to half the blindness in the world (currently around 50 million people) yet if action is taken, it seems to be the easiest of eye problems to heal.

People aged 50 to 90 are being healed by taking minerals, herbs and vitamins.

However a warning – because all these things are deficiency problems, they can return (and have) if some maintenance programme is not continued.

What should I take for cataracts, glaucoma and macular problems?

40% less Cataracts with Lutein and vitamins

British ophthalmologist Dr Evans, a man who has healed eye troubles with minerals and vitamins, quotes a US trial reported in the British Medical Journal in 1992, involving 50,000 nurses over a 10 year period.

It showed that the nurses who had a regular intake of Lutein (an anti-oxidant found mainly in dark leafy vegetables) plus Vitamin A and Vitamin C, had a 40% less chance of developing cataracts than people not taking these essential nutrients.

The report estimated that if Americans could be persuaded to increase their use of just those three substances, Medicare could reduce its budget by 12% due to reduced spending on cataract operations.

Of course, for ophthalmologists to publicise those findings would mean a nasty fall in their income. It would be like asking turkeys to compete in a competition to see who could be first into the oven.

Little research

Because so few medical establishments do any research into the effects of minerals, vitamins and herbs on eye health, most medical treatment is done without the benefit of coordinated research.

Dr Evans' recommendations

Let's look at what Dr Evans recommends that we take daily to prevent or heal cataracts. (The variable amounts depend on how bad the cataracts are.)

70 grams	Protein (minimum) per day.
25,000 to 175,000 iu	Vitamin A as beta carotene.
5 to 15 mg	Vitamins B1, B2, and B6*.
1000 mg	Vitamin B12.

---

* Vitamin B6 is a brain stimulant, and too much can prevent deep sleep, so reduce intake if sleep problems occur. Normal RDI is 1.5 mg a day.

500 to 5000 mg	Vitamin C.
300 to 3000 mg	Vitamin D.
100 to 400mg	Vitamin E.

In addition he suggests to also take Inositol, Potassium, Magnesium, Pantothenic acid, Calcium lactate, Choline, Folate (Folic acid) and Paraminobenzoic acid.

What his success rate was I do not know, but many almost blind cases were healed.

Dr Price-Todd's recommendations

Now compare Dr Evans' treatment with US ophthalmologist Dr Price-Todd, who claims an 88% success rate.

Posterior Sub-capsular cataracts.

2 GTF Chromium tablets for 30 days.
4 Multi-vitamin tablets daily.

Opalescent, Early, and Cortical Spoking cataracts.

4 Multi-vitamin tablets daily.

Brunescent cataracts.

4 Multi-vitamin tablets daily.

For 6 to 12 months take daily:

200 mg	L-Glutathione.
600 mcg	Selenium daily for 12 months.
100 to 300 mg	Vitamin E.
1000 mg	Vitamin C.

Corneal Guttata cataracts.

150 mg CoQ10 for 3 months.
4 Multi-vitamin tablets daily.

Nuclear Sclerosis cataracts.

4 Multi-vitamin tablets daily.

Plus for one year take daily:

200 mg	Glutathione.
600 mg	Selenium.
100 to 300 mg	Vitamin E.
1000 mg	Vitamin C.

Now compare the great differences

There are great differences in what both these eye specialists recommend. The treatments are not even closely similar, yet they both heal.

But note, neither of them suggest herbs, anti-oxidants or Omega 3 oils, all of which, according to latest research, are essential for eye health.

So if I have cataracts what should I take?

Well, in the light of latest research that suggests too much Vitamin B2 can make the eye light-sensitive, this is what I would take as a daily dosage:

2	Multi-vitamin tablets.
200 mg	Vitamin E.
150 mg	CoQ10.
75,000 iu	Vitamin A as beta carotene.
400 mcg	GTF Chromium.
1000 mg	Vitamin C.
600 mg	Omega 3 Flax Seed oil.
100 mg	Ginkgo Biloba extract.
200 mcg	Selenium.
200 mg	Pycnogenol with protectors.
3	Digestive Enzyme supplements. To ensure absorption. One per meal.

In addition, I would take note of Dr Evans' advice and have a minimum protein intake of 70 grams daily. Also try to eat at least one cup of spinach or other dark-leafed vegetable a day.

What should I take for Glaucoma?

For glaucoma I would take all of the above plus:

6 tablets	Perfect Eyes
100 mg	Bilberry extract

For Macular or worse troubles I would also include

4	Multi-mineral tablets.
400 mg	Magnesium (if not in the multi).
400 mg	Potassium (if not in the multi).

5000 mg Lecithin (anti-oxidant).
600 mg Omega 3 fish oil capsules.
3000 mg Taurine (an amino acid).
200 mg Ginkgo Biloba extract

How long before I see results?

Well for cataracts, if you have had no improvement after 7 months, give up.

For glaucoma, if pressures are not down within 2 months, give it away.

For dry or wet macular troubles it could actually take one year before improvement occurs, although minor improvements can occur at 3 or 6 month intervals.

On taking tablets

Some people have difficulty taking tablets and capsules, and you will have many to take, especially in the initial stages where you may be taking 12 or more Pycnogenol alone, besides others.

Health supplement companies, such as Nature Sunshine whom I deal with, also market digestive enzyme supplements such as Proactazyme. These help promote stomach enzymes to aid in quickly assimilating tablets and can help people who claim tablets give them constipation. Plenty of water helps too.

I always take my tablets with meals. I chew a mouthful of food ready to swallow, and then pop in a couple of tablets, mixing them into my food with my tongue. It is no trouble to swallow them.

On using Pycnogenol for all eye conditions

The strong anti-oxidant Pycnogenol is normally sold in 50 mg tablets. The dosage when using it for eye problems is as follows.

1st day Take two tablets per day.
2nd day Take four tablets per day.
3rd day Take six tablets per day.

And so on until you are taking one tablet per day for each stone (6.5 kilograms) you weigh.

So if you weighed 12 stone (76 kg) you would increase

your dosage daily by two tablets until you were taking twelve tablets a day. Stay at this dosage for 14 days, after which you drop off the dosage by two tablets a day until you are back down to four tablets a day (200 mg). Continue at that dosage from then onwards.

Higher potency Pycnogenol available

Remember, you will still be taking the other tablets at the same time. If you have difficulty taking so many, a higher potency 200 mg tablet of Pycnogenol may suit you better.

Being four times stronger, you would start with one, then two, then three, keep that up for two weeks then drop back to one per day from there onwards.

Suggestions on the cost of the treatment

One final suggestion on the cost of the treatment. If you are paying medical insurance and the premiums are keeping you poor, and you have been paying it for years and are approaching 65 and developing eye troubles, consider this:

Next year they will bump up your premium. So do not risk blindness by depriving your eyes of help now because you cannot afford it. Next year your sight may be worse, and you will not be able to afford to pay your premium anyway.

By becoming a member of Nature Sunshine Products at a cost of $20, you can receive up to 30% discount off the retail price of their products which are quite reasonably priced.

Becoming a member does not mean you have to load yourself up with a $1000 worth of products, or even $20 worth of products. But it does mean you can buy their products at a discount.

Signs of mineral imbalance

You can overdose on Selenium, especially on the non-organic selenate type, but I have taken 500 mcg during one day with no sign of an overdose.

The signs of Selenium overdose are: numb or tingling hands or feet, bad breath with a garlic-like odour, brittle nails, hair loss and reddish skin pigmentation.

Unless numbness and tingling happen within four hours of taking it, Selenium is not the cause.

An overdose of Fluoride can give the same sensation, but more likely the cause would be one of the following: A shortage of Calcium, Magnesium or Vitamin B1, B6, or B12.

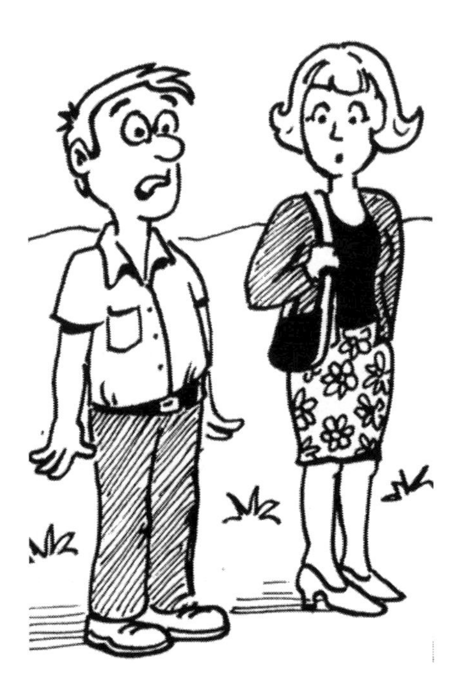

"I'll have to see an eye specialist. I keep seeing spots before my eyes."

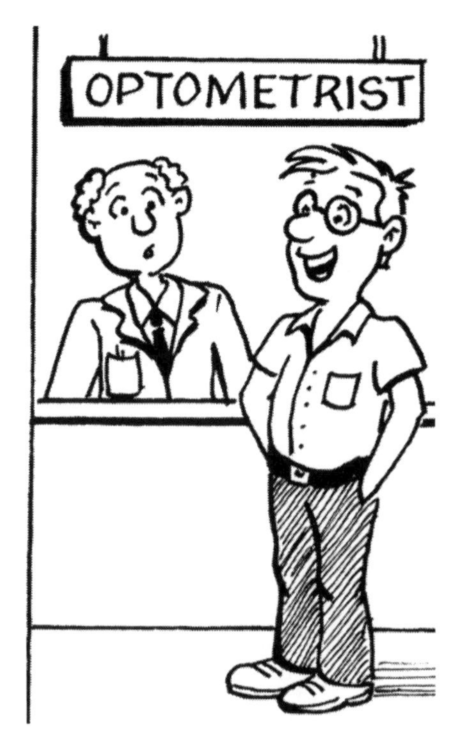

"Wow! That's better! The spots are much clearer now!"

Retinitis Pigmentosa

What is Retinitis Pigmentosa?

Retinitis Pigmentosa or RP is a condition of the eye that gradually progresses to blindness. In most cases slowly, but in some cases quite quickly.

Normally it is a slow, progressive trouble that rarely develops before middle age.

The outer vision is always the first to go and central vision last. Some sufferers have described as like looking through a straw. The common nickname is Tunnel Vision. See the cover picture.

What causes it?

A narrowing of the tiny network of veins in the eye is always the first sign of Retinitis Pigmentosa.

A normal eye contains hundreds of thousands of cells that collect foreign particles and used material, and pass this waste out into the network of these veins for disposal.

In cases of Retinitis Pigmentosa, these tiny veins and channels become clogged with this debris, and the incoming blood cannot freely deliver nourishment to the cells.

Vision loss commences. The first warning the average person will have in most cases is a loss of night vision.

Sometimes these tiny veins and capillaries swell. This condition is called Macular Edema.

Can anything be done?

Well, if you regard your eye specialist as a god who speaks the ultimate truth, then nothing at all can be done.

Some specialists will suggest scatter laser treatment. But this, even if it is successful (and it only helps a few) is only a very short-term help.

Their best advice is usually, "Just prepare to go blind."

Some people, more aware of the very important part minerals and vitamins play in good health, and not prepared to suffer blindness without exploring every avenue, have proved their ophthalmologists to be quite deficient in up-to-date knowledge, especially of alternative treatments.

They still retain their vision. And others who have lost

their vision, by persevering, have actually regained their sight by the use of herbs, minerals and vitamins.

I am willing to try anything; what can I do?

Well, the first thing to do is to try and gain some understanding as to why health disorders occur in our bodies.

Many diseases are caused by fungi, bacteria, or viruses. When these enemies attack a healthy body it musters its resources and fights back. But when they attack a body lacking in minerals and vitamins, they find it much easier to establish a foothold and can be extremely hard to dislodge.

In the course of their occupation, which may last a lifetime, they can cause much pain and disability.

Do these enemies cause eye problems?

No, almost never. There are one or two parasites not found in New Zealand that burrow into eyes and cause discomfort and blindness, but unless someone has been overseas they are not a problem.

Minor bacterial infections such as conjunctivitis can be banished inside one day by bathing the eye in a Colloidal Silver solution. Viral infections may take longer.

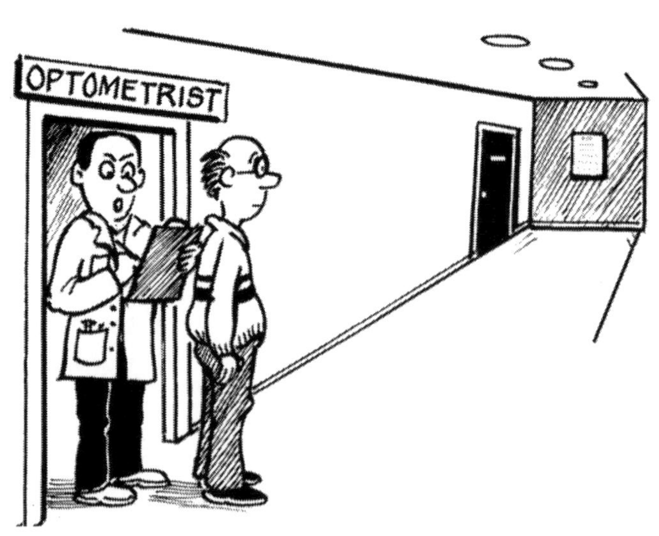

"Wrong! Wrong! Wrong! Wrong! Sorry! You'll have to see my brother-in-law who's a specialist. His office is down there by the eye chart."

What is Colloidal Silver?

Colloidal Silver is one of the safest organism killers ever discovered or used and is totally harmless to humans.

Properly made, Colloidal Silver is pure distilled water to which silver is added by a process of electrolysis. I make it at a ratio of 6 parts silver per million parts of water (6 ppm). I drink it. I spray my vegetables with it.

Long ago, before the days of antibiotics, early American settlers had learned to keep their milk from spoiling during hot summer days and nights. They did this by placing in it a pure silver dollar. These people knew nothing about bacteria, but they did know from experience that a silver dollar in their milk kept it from going sour.

Back in 1910, Dr Henry Crooks, a leader in Colloidal Silver experiments wrote this regarding the effects of Colloidal Silver, *'Bronchial TB, staphylococcus pyogenes, various streptococcus and other pathogenic organisms are all killed in three to four minutes. In fact no microbe is known that is not killed by Colloidal Silver in six minutes, at a concentration of 25 parts per million.'*

Modern research now suggests that a 5 parts per million (ppm) concentrate is ample to kill almost everything, and indeed, concentrations as low as 3 ppm are adequate to kill most organisms.

Colloidal Silver now known to kill over 650 viral, fungal or bacterial organisms

I will go through the alphabet naming just two from each letter: acne, athletes foot, blood parasites, boils, candida, colitis, dermatitis, dysentery, eczema, gonorrhoea, gastritis, hay fever, herpes, impetigo, indigestion, keratosis, leukemia, lupus, malaria, meningitis, neurasthenia, parasite infections, psoriasis, pneumonia, rhinitis, ringworm, shingles, septicaemia, tuberculosis, tonsillitis, ulcers (all forms), warts, whooping cough, yeast infections.

Why haven't we heard about Colloidal Silver?

Some doctors were recognising the value of Colloidal

Silver in the 1930's as an effective germ killer. The problem was that drug companies could not patent it. It was only silver and water.

It was also costly to produce and buy. One ounce of Colloidal Silver cost about $125 and the knowledge of how to make it was limited.

It was legalised as a medicine by the United States Food and Drug Administration around 1936 and that qualification still applies.

The trouble was that in the 1940's antibiotics came into use. Unlike Colloidal Silver, these could be patented. There were big profits in them, and they were much cheaper than Colloidal Silver to use at the time.

Today of course, anyone, any hospital, could make Colloidal Silver, and that is the problem. It is too cheap.

I with my pocket sized silver generator, can manufacture in two hours a whole litre of Colloidal Silver, for a cost of about $1. There is no profit in it compared to an expensive antibiotic.

The serious burns departments of major hospitals in America use silver, as part of a sulphur antibiotic because it is head and shoulders above other substances for healing burns by destroying any harmful bacteria in the burn tissue.

It is also being increasingly used to kill the harmful bacteria in swimming pools and in aircraft water systems.

I doubt if most doctors in New Zealand even know of the existence of Colloidal Silver, let alone what it can do to quickly heal so many complaints.

Will it kill bad breath?

Whether it is caused by bacteria in the mouth or throat, just rinse your mouth with it, swallow it and the bacteria will swan off.

How safe is it?

Colloidal silver made correctly at 6 parts per million is extremely safe. Three teaspoons a day is generally all that is required.

I usually drink a 350 ml glass a day, and have been doing

so for about a year with absolutely no side effects.

Some who drink over a glass a day may find some good bacteria killed in the digestive system and may need to take some acidophilus yoghurt to re-establish good bacteria that might be killed, but I have never had an inkling of any such need.

I know of people who have drunk three cups a day to wipe out the Helicobacter pylori bacteria that cause stomach ulcers, and they have eradicated it smartly, and did not need to take yoghurt afterwards. But perhaps some people may need it.

Cannot harm a day old baby

Colloidal silver can be sprayed into the eye of a day old baby. It is totally harmless. There is no stinging. It can be sprayed in ears, on cuts or rashes, or in the groin, without any stinging or ill effects.

Is it totally harmless under all circumstances?

Yes. You can take as much as you like, provided you use common sense. A concentration of six parts per million (6 ppm), or even half that strength will kill most fungi, bacteria or viruses.

But if you have perhaps a nasty virus that resists that concentration, then by all means use 10 ppm or even 15 ppm.

Have you been personally healed yourself?

Yes. This is one of the ways I got involved with Colloidal Silver. I had bad conjunctivitis which no antibiotic could heal. A friend sprayed my eyes with Colloidal Silver three times in half an hour, and the trouble went in under four hours.

Another way of dealing with conjunctivitis, ulcers behind the eye, or swollen eye tissues is to fill an eye bath, raise it to your eye, blink your eye and roll your eye to allow the Colloidal Silver to kill germs and viruses.

Do the same with the other eye. For as long as you like. It is only harmful to viruses, fungi or bacteria.

For a cold or flu, breathe it into your lungs

There is a very sound reason for breathing atomised Colloidal Silver into your lungs. Firstly it is the quickest way to get Colloidal Silver into your bloodstream. The area of tissue in your lungs exposed to air when you take a deep breath, if laid flat, would cover an area of two football fields.

Breathing it in a vapour or spraying some under your tongue and holding it there for a minute also allows a quick entry of Colloidal Silver to the bloodstream.

Where do I get a sprayer to do that?

I have found an excellent vaporiser sprayer that is ideal for the job. It is in a brown bottle. It is sold in chemist shops and is used to deliver a drug for nasal problems called 'Beconase Aqueous' You may know of someone who uses it regularly and throws the old bottle away.

If you cannot get a bottle that way, buy a bottle. It will cost about $24. Tip the contents down the sink. Wash it thoroughly and fill it with Colloidal Silver. Being a brown glass bottle is good, as light deteriorates Colloidal Silver and it should always be stored in darkness.

You can also buy low cost plastic spray containers made from high grade plastic from a plastics shop. However these are invariably clear and need to be protected from light. This can be done by sticking black insulation tape around the outside.

But be sure you buy a sprayer that produces a fine mist. Some of them are not very good in this respect.

Why store Colloidal Silver in darkness?

The reason is because atoms of silver oxidise in the light.

Colloidal Silver should also never be stored in a fridge, or near a microwave, TV, or any electrical appliances. Reason? Atoms of Colloidal Silver carry a small electrical charge and float suspended in the water. If a magnetic field destroys that charge, they could sink to the bottom of the bottle.

Plastics and Colloidal Silver

Colloidal Silver is best stored in glass.

However PET and HDPE high grade plastics are now being

used for storing Colloidal Silver. This is the grade of plastic used for bottles in the food industry. These high grade plastics are also known as No 1 and No 2 plastic.

Colloidal Silver should never be stored in cheaper grade plastics than this as it can be contaminated by chemicals leaching out of the plastic.

Trying a different approach

If I was suffering and getting no relief from any of those nasties such as lupus, etc, I would not hesitate to spray that fine vapour down my throat and breathe it into my lungs at least three or four times a day.

For confirmation of the efficacy of Colloidal Silver against incurables, get onto the Internet, go into Google or any other search engine, and ask questions about Colloidal Silver. You will be swamped with testimonials.

Should I take supplements as well?

Yes, definitely. In addition to Colloidal Silver I recommend you take major quantities of minerals, vitamins, herbs and anti-oxidants.

Nowadays, with depleted soils and the use of chemical fertilisers, these things are essential for eye and body health.

Where can I buy Colloidal Silver?

Colloidal Silver is available in most health shops. If you wish to obtain some to spray into your mouth or up your nostrils to kill a cold, or stop a sore throat in its tracks, it is excellent source for that purpose. Try some.

But if you wished to use it on a more extensive scale, such as I do, you will need plenty of cash to buy it in this way. I recommend you make it yourself cheaply by buying a generator.

Are we really short of minerals and vitamins?

Let's get away from eyes, to sheep for a moment. I am a retired farmer myself.

In 1938, a devastating sickness struck many New Zealand sheep flocks – facial eczema. The skin peeled from their faces and they suffered agonising pain until death.

From that time onwards, whenever moist humid conditions followed summer dryness, the disease reappeared.

Our Government employed scientists to discover the cause. Eventually after decades of research, at a cost of millions of dollars, a great announcement was made and honours bestowed. The 'cause' of facial eczema had been found. Fungal spores that the sheep ingested under certain conditions were the culprits.

Now that the 'cause' had been found, the next thing was how to deal with these spores. This was a time of joy for the animal pharmaceutical firms. They produced a fungicide that farmers purchased in huge quantities and sprayed onto their land to kill the spores. A costly business, but it worked.

An observant and intelligent woman

While the scientists were busy with their research, one farmer's wife, who felt extreme sympathy for the suffering of her sheep, tried salving their peeled, burnt faces with zinc ointment.

It immediately soothed the pain and speeded up the healing. She wondered if it was perhaps a shortage of Zinc that was the prime cause of facial eczema.

She was correct. Sheep given a Zinc drench, or living off pastures topdressed with Zinc, rarely developed eczema.

Nowadays no farmer sprays his pasture with fungicide to treat facial eczema, they include Zinc with their fertilisers or drench their sheep with Zinc.

So lets get back to eyes

Some financially-supported eye researchers are adamant that most eye disorders have a genetic cause and eye deterioration is inevitable.

Others, mainly self-financed, are not so convinced and give serious consideration to a lack of minerals, vitamins, bioflavonoids, enzymes and hormones as possibly the prime cause of the so-called incurable eye troubles.

When we are young, our bodies manufacture all the hormones and enzymes that we need. But as we age we no longer produce them in the amounts needed, and must supplement if we wish to keep good vision.

This also poses a question – if the eye disorders considered incurable, such as Cataracts, Retinitis Pigmentosa, Macular Degeneration and Glaucoma, are due to genetic factors, then please explain how numerous people using natural supplements have been healed?

Having myself seen and heard of so many people lowering eye pressures and recovering sight by means of taking natural supplements, I can only say to all eye sufferers – if you can afford it, give it a try. How much is your sight worth to you?

The missing elements

Afflictions like blood pressure, gall stones, PMS, osteoporosis, heart troubles, aneurisms, varicose veins and dozens of other ailments, do not have any origin in bacteria, fungal activity, or viruses. They are symptoms of a serious shortage of the essential elements necessary to good health.

Diseases, fungal, viral, or bacterial, unless they are of a particularly virulent type, can only attack and gain a hold in an unhealthy body. But where the body's defences have been kept at full strength, via supplements of minerals, vitamins, herbs, enzymes, etc, disease finds it very hard to win the battle.

While pharmaceutical drugs or the surgeons knife may seem an easy way to remove ills from our bodies, body parts cannot be cut away forever, and medical drugs often produce severe side effects.

Expensive urine?

The sarcastic comment of many in the medical profession that people who supplement on vitamins have very expensive urine, has as much validity as the ancient tale that the stork delivered babies.

No urine is more expensive than that from patients on medical prescription drugs, sometimes four or five of them, all with side effects, often acting against one another, and often removing valuable minerals from our bodies.

They can be well over a hundred times more expensive than minerals and vitamins, and often with little or no satisfaction.

Side effects of prescription drugs in just one year, in 1995 in the USA, cost around $76,000,000,000 dollars in extra medical care costs.

Now that's what I call expensive urine.

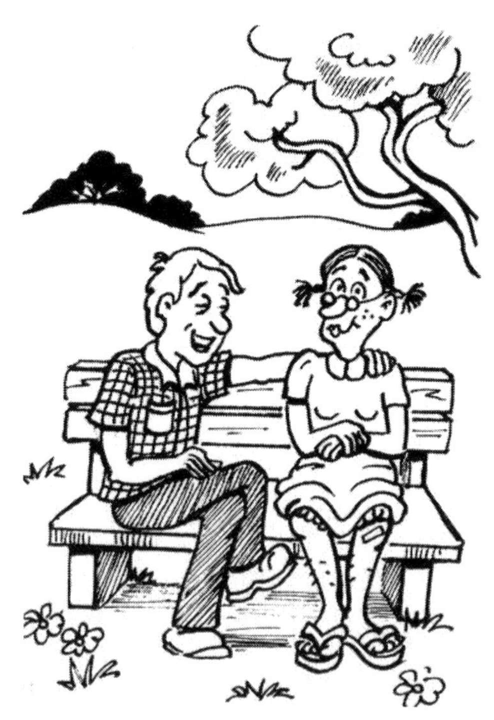

"The doc reckons my eyes need seeing to! But it doesn't stop me picking up a pretty girl!"

The liver – our body's warehouse

If our eyes could leave our body at will and sit on a pole at their leisure, they could be treated as separate entities. But they cannot leave. They are a vital part of our body. And if our eyes are not well, neither is our body.

If our eyes are short of minerals, so are our bodies. We cannot take Selenium and instruct our bodies to just deliver it to our eyes. Our heart may need it more urgently, even though we may not be aware of that fact.

If we are to enjoy good health, then the old false belief that bodily parts can be individually treated must give way to the more sensible approach of holistic treatment

Blood – our cell's delivery service.

Healthy blood is essential to a healthy body. It acts as a delivery service to the cells, supplying what is needed to all parts.

The nutrient warehouse of our body is the liver.

The liver stores our vitamins, enzymes, steroids, etc. Some of these our liver has manufactured itself, some have been delivered to it.

When supplies are surplus to requirements, they are stored in the liver warehouse. If we starve for a couple of months, our liver will keep sending supplies on demand until it runs out of product.

But whether we eat or starve, if we do not in the first place deliver to the warehouse all the essential things our bodies need to stay healthy, they cannot be delivered to parts that need them.

The liver is also a nutrient manufacturer

Besides acting as a central warehouse, our liver also manufactures, stores or delivers steroids, acids, bioflavonoids, enzymes, hormones and fatty vitamins A, E, and D. Here are some important ones.

DHEA (Dehydro-epi-androsterone) DHEA is a hormone manufactured by our adrenal gland. It appears to counter the effects of excess cortisol released during times of stress and is regarded as an essential anti-aging hormone.

It is widely sold over the counter in many countries including America as a wonderful anti-aging product.

When Natures Sunshine Products attempted to introduce this natural hormone into New Zealand in 1997, our government banned it. Perhaps they were concerned that too many New Zealanders would survive too long on superannuation.

Cortisol Cortisol is a powerful hormone, manufactured by the adrenal gland. It is vital for many functions in our bodies and in particular, to cope with stressful situations.

Cortisol and DHEA tend to balance one another. As we age it seems that more cortisol is produced and it becomes dominant.

High levels of Cortisol have been linked with many diseases, including alcoholism, drug abuse, anorexia, Alzheimer's, diabetes, hypertension, all forms of cancer, strokes, heart attacks, psoriasis and many others.

At the time of writing, to the best of my knowledge no method has yet been devised to measure when Cortisol levels are too high. It is always safer to have too much DHEA than too much Cortisol.

Taurine An amino acid and anti-oxidant. When injected intravenously it can bring major improvement to Macular Degeneration. Oral doses of 2 or 3 grams daily can be helpful. It is also useful in some Retinitis Pigmentosa cases.

Taurine protects the retina against sunlight and acts as a booster for the enzyme Glutathione (see below).

CoQ10 A very powerful anti-oxidant and anti-aging enzyme. Some eye researchers believe it can substitute for Vitamin E. It can markedly reduce blood pressure and is always deficient in people with heart problems.

Sardines, baked beans and eggs are a good source of raw CoQ from which a healthy liver makes CoQ10. Mice fed CoQ10 have added 50% to their normal life span.

As we age our liver loses the ability to manufacture it in sufficient quantity. When we drop below 25% of what was normal in our bodies to fight disease, we die.

Glutathione This enzyme is manufactured in our body cells and stored and delivered by the liver. Glutathione needs sulphur-rich foods such as eggs, onions, garlic and asparagus to be made inside the body but can be obtained naturally from avocado, watermelon, asparagus and grapefruit.

It is another powerful anti-oxidant. People with low levels of Glutathione in the blood are much more subject to disease.

Lutein In the centre of the retina is a yellow pigment called Lutein. It is a very important anti-oxidant which protects the eye from sunlight damage.

Smokers and post-menopausal women have only half the normal requirement of Lutein, and carry a greater risk of serious eye trouble. Tests on animals deprived of Lutein showed a rapid development of eye problems.

Lutein is only needed in micro amounts but is extremely hard to absorb. It is found in all dark green leafy vegetables but the very best source is kale. This green vegetable appears to have twice as much as any other plant.

One person who ate a cup of kale per day for one year regained 50% of his vision lost to Wet Macular Degeneration. Between 20 mg to 40 mg is a good supplement if you cannot eat a cup of kale per day.

Lutein always works in the company of Zeaxanthin which is a Vitamin A like carotenoid pigment.

The suggested dosage of Lutein is 40 mg daily for two months, then dropping to 20 mg per day. Always leave a gap of 7 hours between taking Vitamin A and Lutein.

Beta Carotene is a close cousin to Lutein and Zeaxanthin. All of these are what is known as bioflavonoids. Beta Carotene is found in all fruits and vegetables, especially in those with orange-coloured flesh, ie, apricots, pumpkin, carrots, etc.

Our body turns it into Vitamin A as required. Most eyes with health problems lack Vitamin A.

Bioflavonoids – your body's police force

In 1968, no doubt spurred on by the drug cartels who don't like people using products they cannot patent, the United States Food and Drug Administration (FDA) declared, "*Bioflavonoids are ineffective for the treatment of any human condition whatsoever.*" It was then banned from any mention in medical prescriptions.

Proanthocyanidin

The bioflavonoid Proanthocyanidin (two popular brands extracted from grape seeds or pine bark are marketed as Pycnogenol and Grapine) is an anti-oxidant that is rapidly becoming known among herbalists as a wonder treatment for many human ailments.

While the medical profession barely knows of its existence and cannot prescribe it, health shops are reporting amazing results with this natural product of grape seed or pine bark.

Proanthocyanidin is essential for the treatment of eyes. It is 20 times more powerful than Vitamin C and 50 times more powerful than Vitamin E. It is both an anti-oxidant and catalyst and reduces the fragility of the tiny veins of the eye. It has been licensed and approved by the medical profession in France as a treatment for Diabetic Retinopathy.

It helps all eye conditions by improving blood flow and capillary permeability and improves the functioning of the retina.

Proanthocyanidin has many other valuable properties pertaining to skin, aging, tumours, brain function, etc. Stories abound about this wonder healer.

What are anti-oxidants?

Oxidation is involved in many disease processes in our human body. Every moment of our lives, cells in the process of living or dying split and give off atoms of oxygen in a process called oxidation. This process of cell division takes place in about a fiftieth of a second or less.

Consider these freed oxygen atoms as desirable young women.

Regard anti-oxidants as an army of young bachelors, seeking wives from among these freed oxygen atoms.

Look upon these young men as our body's anti-oxidant police force, stationed along the thousands of kilometres of our blood highway to protect us from harm.

For also stationed along our blood highway, are criminal characters like cancer and other disease-causing organisms.

They too are seeking to capture some of these desirable young women (oxygen atoms), because without them they cannot increase.

The larger the number of the anti-oxidant police force, the less the chances the baddies have of raising a family.

So far, scientists have discovered over 20,000 anti-oxidants in nuts, fruits and other plants.

Keep your anti-oxidant police force at full strength

Saturate your blood with anti-oxidants and almost all disease organisms die of starvation.

But if your blood highway is not saturated with anti-oxidants, these very desirable oxygen atoms escape from both the good and the bad who seek them and strike up damaging relationships every day with thousands of healthy cells.

Who are the members of this anti-oxidant police force ?

Well they come in all shapes and sizes, but the most important, or shall we say the police commissioners, are called anthocyanidin bioflavonoids. This bioflavonoid is 20 times more powerful than Vitamin C and 50 times more powerful than Vitamin E. It is also found in elderberry, huckleberry, bilberry and cranberry.

Other different bioflavonoids are found in red onions, red apples, cherries, red beet, lemons, oranges and limes and the bark of most shrubs and trees. In fact all vegetables and fruit contain some bioflavonoids.

Enzymes and foot soldiers are both needed

Among the police on the beat along the blood highway army, we find two important enzymes made by our body, especially when we are young and healthy. These are CoQ10 and Glutathione.

Both these enzymes are manufactured by and stored in our liver. But as we age, we lose the ability to make them in sufficient quantities. Glutathione cannot perform properly without the assistance of Selenium and Sulphur.

Also important among the police we could name Selenium, Zinc, Beta Carotene, Folic acid, Vitamins A, C, E, and P.

What you ask is Vitamin P? Well in the days when it was found that Vitamin C cured scurvy, it did not cure all scurvy. The only thing that could cure haemorrhagic scurvy was a substance found in lemon juice. At the time it was called Vitamin P. Later it lost that title to be called a bioflavonoid.

How else do anti-oxidants help?

They have the ability to allow the blood to travel through the tiniest veins in our bodies, to re-open blocked blood vessels and allow the blood to nourish cells and carry away waste products.

An example of this is the hundreds of millions of night vision cells in our eyes called rods. These use Vitamin A in the process of seeing in the dark.

In the morning light, this used-up Vitamin A is pushed out into the bloodstream to be carted away. If those tiny blood capillaries become blocked, they swell (a condition called edema) and vision loss occurs.

So you can see that anti-oxidants are very important to our bodies, especially our eyes.

Why extra oxygen can help

It has been found that people who have suffered a stroke or heart attack, and who also have Retinitis Pigmentosa, and are given emergency 100% oxygen treatment to breathe in controlled doses, notice an immediate improvement to their eyes and brain. This is because of the increased oxygen content of their impaired blood supply.

However this extra oxygen intake also increases the oxidation of cells, so it is important when breathing pure oxygen, to saturate your blood with anti-oxidants – bioflavonoids, Vitamin C, Zinc, Selenium, CoQ10, etc, to counter this.

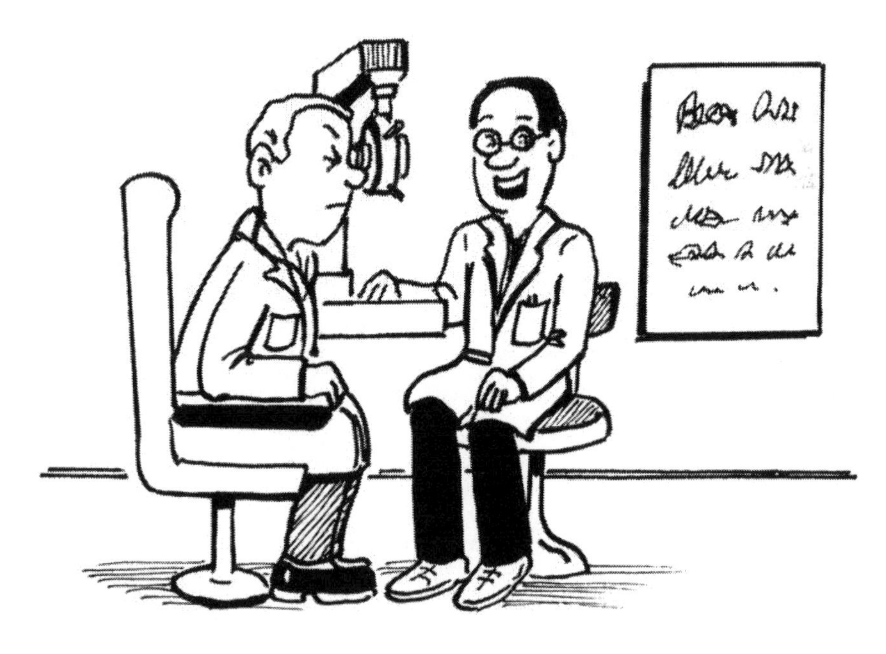

"As you're a doctor, we have a special eye chart for you."

Other facts about eyes

Medical drugs lower your chance of eye improvement

From reports I have received, it is a fact that people who are on drugs supplied by drug companies, via their doctor, have a far lower chance of eye improvement than those who take no medical drugs.

For example, a study on nutrition for the aged by an American university found that many pharmaceutical drugs block vital nutritional uptake, and the longer they are taken, the greater the risk of nutritional side effects.

Deficiency in one nutrient can cause a side effect, which most doctors, because they know so little about minerals or vitamins, will then attempt to cure by prescribing another drug which may even cause more damage.

Side effects of medical drugs

There are over 60 medical drugs that rob the body of essential nutrients, particularly the eyes. The commonly prescribed pills for stomach acidity (Losec, etc), and laxatives deplete Vitamin A, D, E, and K. And aspirin destroys Vitamin C.

Latest American research suggests that over one quarter of all drugs currently prescribed to the elderly can cause unhealthy side effects.

A 1990 American study found 40% of doctor's patients aged over 65 took an average of five prescription drugs daily, and another 19% took seven drugs daily.

This mixing of drugs can cause many problems. Among them, dizziness, bladder trouble and mental disorientation.

People who have high blood pressure and take Valium can develop severe mental problems.

Arthritic drugs react badly with alcohol and coffee to the detriment of the stomach.

Heart medications used along with a diuretic, can intensify the side effects of each drug. Also statin-type cholesterol-lowering drugs such as Lipex hinder the liver from making CoQ10.

The blood-thinner Warfarin (also a rat poison) combined with aspirin can cause internal bleeding, and has done so in eyes, causing blindness.

The desired effects of diabetic and asthma drugs can be negated by some eyedrops, and conversely the drugs in some eyedrops can bring on asthma and/or heart trouble.

So you see, if people on doctor's drugs use herbs, minerals and vitamin supplements and get no relief for eye problems, it is not surprising.

For children with weak eyes, try Zinc with Vitamin C and Bilberry.

Avoid these drugs or substances – they are deadly for eyes

This is not a final list. I have no doubt there are many more.

MSG 621 (Monosodium Glutamate) This toxic flavour enhancer is widely used in the food industry to make inferior savoury foods, such as soups, sauces and processed meats taste better and to keep greens looking fresh.

MSG in high doses is a powerful nerve and brain toxin (excitotoxin) that can damage brain and nerve cells, creating serious mental and body symptoms.

But MSG is such a great flavour enhancer and works so well at disguising off-tastes from poor ingredients, that it is just too tempting for most manufacturers not to use MSG in their products. But because it has a bad name in the public eye you will often see the MSG listed as 'flavour enhancer' 'natural flavours' or 'yeast extracts' on most products. MSG lurks everywhere, even in health products. Buyer beware.

Oils/fats heated over 100°C during manufacturing

These include all margarines, corn oil, safflower oil, canola oil, all hydrogenated fats. These become unnatural oils with toxic effects and should be avoided.

Exjade/Deferasirox A medical drug to remove excess Iron from the body. Causes blind spots, colour problems, blurred vision, and night blindness by removing minerals from the blood.

Ethambutol Similar effect to Exjade. Removes minerals.

Plaquenil Also removes minerals. Night blindness and pigment changes.

Aspartame 951 See special chapter on Aspartame.

Prednisone and Cortisone Both of these remove Zinc, one of the most essential minerals for your eyes and whole body and widely deficient in almost all world populations.

Here are just a few of the 30 or more disorders arising from lack of Zinc – high cholesterol, weak blood cells, lack of energy, arthritis, prostate troubles, high blood pressure, failing sight.

Tamoxifen A deadly drug, that is supposed to repel breast cancer, but is actually useless for that purpose.

6% of women taking this virulent uterus and liver cancer-forming drug suffer decreased vision and damage to the retina and cornea. And at 40 mg per day they can suffer irreversible corneal and retinal changes. Eyes not suffering immediate vision loss may be predisposed to later problems.

In 1995 the State of California Carcinogen Identification Committee unanimously voted to add Tamoxifen to its list! Many doctors still prescribe this deadly and useless drug to New Zealand women with breast cancer.

Penicillamine Causes skin disorders, loss of eyelashes. retinal pigment changes and is under suspicion of promoting Retinitis Pigmentosa.

Thiazide A combination of diuretics that removes body minerals.

Phenothiazine tranquilliser Also a diuretic that removes body minerals.

Psoralens, Melleril, Stelazine, Chlorpromazine All these are under suspicion of causing eye problems.

Tobacco and Nicotine Bad for the total body, including the eyes.

Olestra fat blocker Removes essential fatty acids and hinders the body's processing of vitamins A, K, E, and D which are essential for the eyes.

Viagra A sex drug that affects eye pigments. No doubt more side effects yet to be discovered.

Caffeine One cup of coffee reduces blood flow to the retina by 13%.

Aspirin As little as 75 mg can cause haemorrhages in the retina. So can non-steroidal anti-inflammatory pain tablets. There is evidence of a strong connection between constant aspirin intake and Macular Degeneration (bleeding in the blood vessels of the retina that cause blindness).

Alcohol Interferes with liver function, reducing the protective levels of glutathione and impairing night vision.

Vigabatrin An epilepsy drug. Causes vision problems.

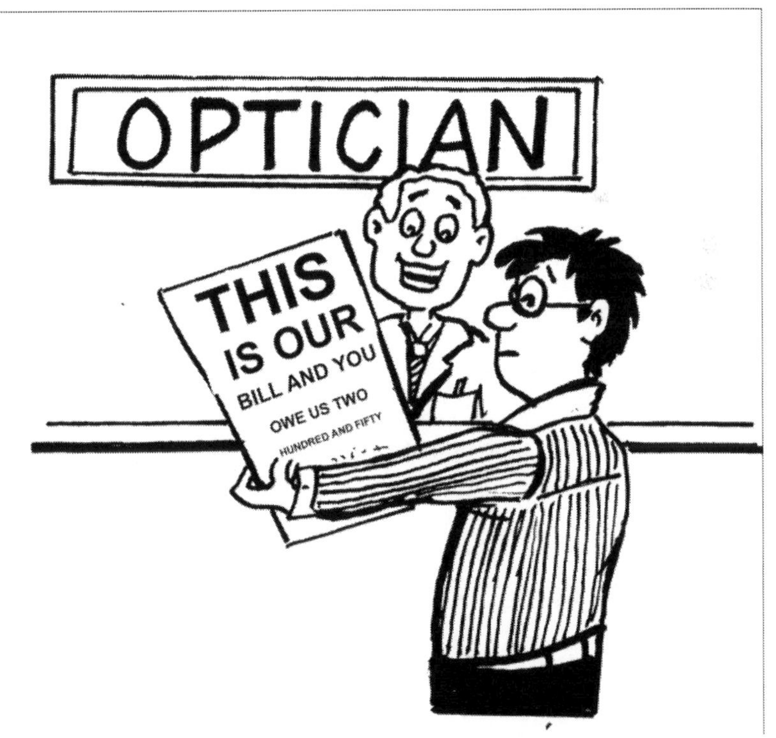

"We think it adds a nice touch sir."

Herbs that help your eyes

Eyebright

The herb eyebright has a history of human usage of over 2000 years. For centuries it has been regarded as a specific remedy for tired, inflamed, or watery eyes.

The flower of the plant has a signature on it that looks like the retina of a human eye, hence the name.

Sap from the plant was anciently described as *'a precious water to clear a man's sight.'*

The writings of a 17th century English herbalist say, *'Indeed, it has a powerful effect to help and restore sight decayed by age.'*

Dr Dorothy Shepherd quotes many cases where prolonged use of eyebright gave very successful results to many eye conditions. She also found the herb useful in the treatment of measles.

In connection with this, a British doctor John Evans writes, *'The plant eyebright has a specific action on the mucous lining of the eye, the nose and the uppermost parts of the throat, as far as the windpipe. Its action on the lachrymal structures of the eye, causing tears to flow, is the prime reason for its use in the case of measles, because it prevents the eye from becoming injured.'*

Ginkgo Biloba

Studies have shown that this extract appears to improve and prevent memory loss but this herb has long been used as a help for eyes. Researchers have now discovered that it gives impressive results in the treatment of Macular Degeneration. It improves the supply of blood and oxygen to the retina and is a good anti-oxidant.

Suggested dosage is 100 mg to 200 mg per day.

Taurine

The amino acid Taurine assists blood to the retina and protects eyes against damage from sunlight. Injected intravenously it can bring major improvement to Macular conditions.

Even an oral dose of 2 to 3 grams daily is very helpful.

Bilberry

The recorded use of Bilberry extends back to the 16th century. Even then it was recognised as helpful to eyes. Recently it has been recognised as a very powerful anti-oxidant.

Anthocyanoside, the active ingredient of Bilberry, stimulates the production of visual purple (rhodopsin). How well we see is directly related to the amount of visual purple we have in the retinal rods of the eye.

A French medical journal published a study by a Dr D. Demure which showed that Bilberry is better than most flavonoids in stopping the breakdown of capillary walls.

In combination with Selenium, Zinc and Vitamin C, Bilberry can reduce clotting of blood every bit as efficiently as aspirin, without the haemorrhaging, macular degeneration and loss of vision associated with aspirin.

Bilberry has tested positive in treating diabetics who develop Glaucoma and Hypertension-caused eye problems. It is excellent for tired eyes.

Dosage 50 mg to 100 mg daily.

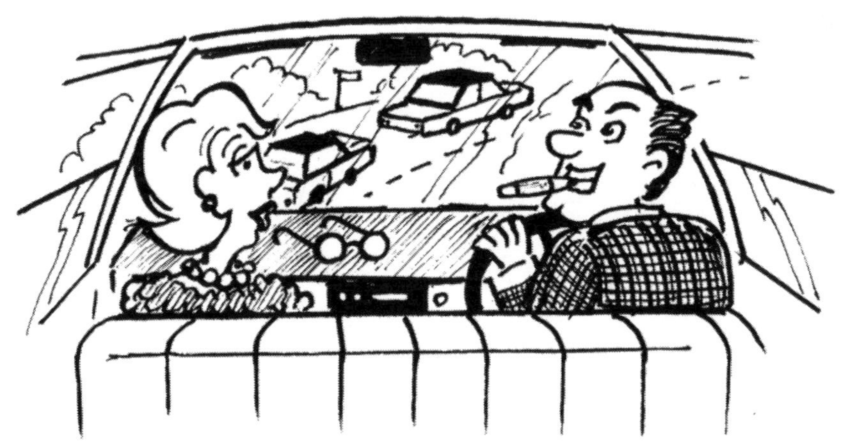

"No, I don't need those glasses for driving. I've had the windscreen ground to my prescription."

Minerals that help your eyes

Zinc

Zinc has been shown to be deficient in almost all the elderly, not to mention many young New Zealanders.

Zinc supplements have been shown to be effective in maintaining good eye health. Adequate Zinc is essential to combat macular degeneration.

Taking over 180 mg of Zinc a day can cause Copper deficiency, but many researchers now suggest, and tests confirm, that people who take about 150 mg of Zinc a day have significant improvement in eyesight, or less loss of vision than those not taking a Zinc supplement.

I repeat, most people do not get enough Zinc in their diets. In a study of 150 people between the ages of 40 and 90, those who took Zinc at 200 mg a day for up to two years had significantly less vision loss than people not on Zinc supplements (Archives of Ophthalmology, Vol.110, P1597, 1992).

Some researchers dispute these findings and say 50 mg a day is adequate. I generally take over 100 mg a day.

Zinc is used by the liver to transport Vitamin A to the eyes and helps remove excess Copper from our system. Too much Zinc could remove the Copper you need for healthy blood, so be sure you have an adequate Copper intake.

Zinc is essential for a healthy prostate in men, and important for the correct functioning of insulin in our bodies. For best absorption, Zinc should be taken on an empty stomach, preferably with a glass of water, about 20 minutes before a meal.

A simple test for Zinc deficiency is to examine your fingernails. If you see white flecks in most of your nails you are probably short of Zinc. A poor sense of taste or smell is also a pointer.

Selenium

New Zealanders are known to be extremely deficient in this important mineral. Tests done in New Zealand in the 1970's showed New Zealanders' blood levels of Selenium to be among the lowest in the world.

A team of American scientists had their blood levels tested when they arrived in New Zealand and also when they left six months later. During that time their Selenium blood levels had dropped by 50%.

Selenium is not only important for eye health, it is essential for all functions of the human body. Australia is supposed to have sufficient Selenium in its soils and foods, but my experience has been that Australians also need to use Selenium with mineral and vitamin supplements to obtain maximum results.

Like Zinc, we just do not get enough Selenium in our foods for good health. Some eye researchers suggest an intake of 200 mg to 400 mg of Selenium daily (dependent on weight) as essential for eye health in the elderly.

Selenium also appears to be essential for blood capillary health. I personally take 300 mcg daily.

The signs of Selenium overdose as mentioned earlier are: numb or tingling hands or feet, bad breath with a garlic-like odour, brittle nails, hair loss and reddish skin pigmentation. Unless numbness and tingling happen within four hours of taking it, Selenium is not the cause.

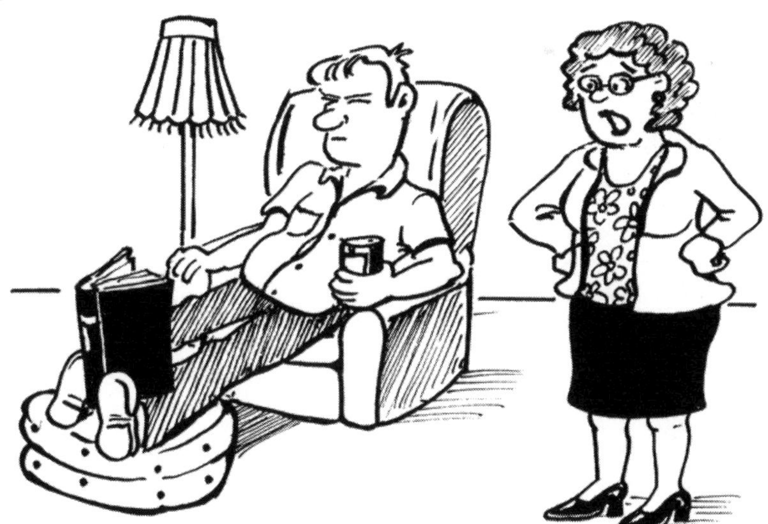

"Oh for heaven's sake Bill, swallow your pride and get glasses!"

Do your eyes lack vitamins?

This much we do know: lack of Vitamin A makes people prone to cataracts, irritable inflamed eyes, and weak night vision.

In some publications you may see Vitamin A referred to as Retinol, because of its association with the retina.

In almost any eye disorder, not enough Vitamin A will be a contributing factor.

It was once thought that too much Vitamin A could cause health problems, but most scientists now agree that any dosage under 100,000 iu of Vitamin A will be quite safe, except in the case of pregnancy, where too much could cause birth defects.

Vitamin A is essential if the eye is to manufacture visual purple, which is essential for night vision.

It is also essential for all mucous membranes, and has long been successfully used as an anti-cancer vitamin.

Modern eye researchers say minor eye problems require 5,000 iu of Vitamin A a day, and major ones could benefit from 20,000 iu a day. However, most eye defects in adults require a minimum daily intake of 60,000 iu.

In fact, British ophthalmologist S. Evans states that in some harder-to-correct eye disorders, up to 160,000 units of beta carotene were used successfully.

You cannot overdose on the beta carotene form of Vitamin A

Vitamin A can be taken in the form of beta carotene, which is stored in the skin, or straight Vitamin A (Retinol).

Beta carotene is found in all fruits and vegetables, especially those with orange-coloured flesh such as carrots, pumpkins and apricots.

It pays to bear in mind that straight Vitamin A (Retinol) cannot be absorbed into the body without essential fatty acids such as Omega 3 oils. Also, straight Vitamin A can be harmful, whereas it is not possible to overdose on beta carotene. Our body turns it to Vitamin A only as required.

In view of this I suggest you use the safer beta carotene, which does not need fatty acids immediately to be absorbed. However research suggests not to take beta carotene at the same meal as green vegetables.

It is worth noting that a healthy liver can store several months' supply of Vitamin A, so provided your intake is adequate, it is not something you need to take daily.

Vitamin A has long been used as an anti-cancer vitamin, especially for treating leukemia, and is also useful to fight acne and skin wrinkles.

A stomach ulcer could signify low absorption of Vitamin A

Researchers are treating with suspicion the Helicobacter pylori bacterium that causes stomach ulcers. They feel it may interfere in the absorption of Vitamin A. And all fat soluble vitamins, especially if there is a lack of Omega fatty acids in the diet.

They feel this interference with the absorption of Vitamin A may be an underlying cause of coronary artery disease, uveitis (eye inflammation), eczema and many other medical problems.

Lack of Vitamin B2 (Riboflavin)

While Vitamin B2 is essential, researchers have now discovered it is a phototoxin. That is, it attracts light photons which can interact unfavourably with the retina.

They suggest that people with eye problems should not take more than 10 mg a day. Some Vitamin B complex supplements have 100mg of Vitamin B2 in them, along with the other B vitamins.

The RDI of Vitamin B2 is less than 2 mg a day. 100mg of B2 is far too much to take.

Lack of Vitamin B5 (Pantothenic acid)

Lack of Vitamin B5 (Pantothenic acid) means weaker vision as we age. This vitamin is found in small amounts in nearly all foods and can also be manufactured by a healthy liver. Low levels are often found in arthritics, which may be due to a poorly functioning liver.

Lamb and beef liver are good food sources.

Lack of Vitamin B6 (Pyridoxine)

Lack of Vitamin B6 (Pyridoxine) means our bodies find it hard to assimilate Zinc or Iron no matter how much is available in our foods. And Zinc is essential for eye health. However too much Vitamin B6 can act as a brain stimulant and interfere with restful sleep. So limit B6 to 15 mg a day, even less if you are not sleeping well. The RDI is around 2 mg a day.

Lack of Vitamin C

This essential vitamin and anti-oxidant is extremely important for many of our bodily functions, especially our eyes.

Our eye cells require ten times more Vitamin C than is found in blood. And 1000 mg a day is needed to saturate our blood. Vitamin C protects our eyes against damage by sunlight.

Vitamin C has also been found essential to control stress. Long term use of 1000 mg a day increases a normal human lifespan by six years, and reduces the chance of developing cataracts by 70%.

On the other hand, one cigarette reduces the Vitamin C in our blood by 25 mg.

Lack of Vitamin D

Lack of Vitamin D can cause cataracts, even in children. While we are still young Vitamin D is manufactured efficiently through the action of sunlight on our skin. But it seems necessary for most people to supplement our intake of Vitamin D as we age.

Lack of Vitamin E

Lack of Vitamin E means an increased chance of cataracts and heart trouble.

Vitamin E is another powerful anti-oxidant, extremely important for the fatty acid membranes that line the photoreceptors of the eye. Like Vitamin A, it is fat-soluble and competes with Vitamin A for fatty acids.

For this reason, modern researchers advise people not to take Vitamin E and A at the same time. Take them eight hours apart from each other. However this reaction does not occur if the beta carotene form of Vitamin A is taken.

Be sure when buying Vitamin E to buy the natural form, not an artificial synthetic. Natural Vitamin E is called d-alpha-tocopherol. The synthetic one manufactured by the Roche drug company is called dl-alpha-tocopherol.

The suggested dosage of Vitamin E for eye health is between 100 mg to 400 mg daily.

Vitamin E, Selenium, chromium and sulphur are an essential combination for the maintenance of the retinal pigment epithelium (RPE), a layer of cells that covers the eyes' photoreceptors.

Omega 3 and essential fatty acids (EFA's)

Essential fatty acids are food oils. There are three of them: Omega 3, Omega 6 and Omega 9. All food oils are a blend of these three.

Omega 3 is highest in fish oils and Flax Seed oil (also known as Linseed oil).

Omega 6 is highest in corn and safflower oils. Omega 9 in olive oil. However it is not wise to have too much of these latter two. Provided we have an adequate intake of Omega 3, our bodies can normally manufacture the others.

Omega 3 is the most essential of all three. From this our body obtains an important acid called Docosahexaenoic acid, or DHA for short.

Nerve cells throughout the body cannot operate efficiently without DHA. It is now believed by many researchers that a lack of DHA is responsible for a great many nerve disorders.

DHA lines 50% of all brain and retinal cells, and lack of it is a common factor in a number of eye complaints.

People with the following 14 health disorders, apart from their eye problems, have noted very considerable improvement by supplementing their diet with Omega 3:

Addictions	Allergies	Viral infections
Arthritis	Diabetes	Dry Skin
Eczema	Psoriasis	Anaemia

Candida	PMS	Heart Problems
Cancer	Multiple Sclerosis	

DHA and your eyes

It's easier to maintain good eye health if our body is healthy. Research has shown the increasing importance to eyes of DHA.

DHA cannot be manufactured in our bodies without Omega 3 oils. Cold pressed Flax Seed oil is an Omega 3 oil which our liver can process into DHA, but the manufacturing process in our liver takes about six weeks.

It can be introduced to our bodies ready-made, by eating salmon, sardines, or some other type of oily fish, or by taking a capsule of Omega 3 oil containing instant DHA.

It is important to search for a product containing more DHA than other brands. It is also very important to try to find one containing Vitamin E.

Do not purchase products containing DHA with sunflower or safflower oils. Such products, even though they contain DHA, are in by far the majority of cases of little use. Something stops the DHA moving to the eyes.

It is not wise to overdose on DHA. Suggested dosage is 1000 mg per day with perhaps 400 mg of Vitamin E.

Why you should take Vitamin E with DHA?

Both Vitamin E and Vitamin A are anti-oxidants and have an affinity for Omega 3 fats. Like all fats, DHA oxidises and casts off free radical atoms of oxygen unless it is prevented from doing so by the anti-oxidant action of these two vitamins. Both Vitamin A and E are called fat-soluble vitamins.

But Vitamin A competes with Vitamin E for absorption and transport to the liver. So always take Vitamin A eight hours apart from DHA and Vitamin E.

Vitamin E is also essential to prevent the oxidation of cells when sunlight strikes the eyes.

Eating fatty foods depletes the body of Vitamin E.

Other eye troubles

Uveitis

Uveitis is an uncommon but very painful complaint. Nerve pains shoot through the eye. Some refer to it as shingles in the eye.

One person I know had this problem and tried all the eye helps, including Pycnogenol, without success.

But anyone who has this problem and has found no help could well try Echinacea and Cats Claw (Uno de Gato). Both these herbs attack this herpes-like virus.

Austrian doctors claim to have healed this condition by use of the herb Cats Claw. They say it took a year to heal the complaint.

It is suspected H. Pylori bacteria in the stomach (yes, the one that causes stomach ulcers) can sometimes cause this condition, due to the non-absorption of essential oils.

In the light of what I know about Colloidal Silver, the first thing I would suggest to use is an eyebath and bathe the eyes in Colloidal Silver. Roll them around to get the liquid behind the eyes.

Conjunctivitis

This is caused by bacteria and signifies its presence by a slimy discharge, especially at night. When you awake in the morning, your eyelids may be stuck together until you rub them. It generally requires an antibiotic in the form of an eye drop to heal.

But many bacteria are now immune to even the most powerful antibiotics. So just buy some Colloidal Silver and an eye bath. Bathe each eye with Colloidal Silver solution for a few minutes and the bacteria will die.

Dry eyes or dry mouth, or both

If this complaint is not caused by diabetes, that's always the first thing to check, or Aspartame (see page 94) you may have a condition called Sjogren's syndrome (pronounced 'show-grins'). A condition not to be taken lightly.

It affects many people over 65 years of age. They can wake

up after midnight with a very dry mouth.

If this happens to you, purchase a bottle of suckable Vitamin C tablets. Keep them by your bed. If you wake up with a dry mouth, pop in a Vitamin C tablet. Saliva will come almost instantly.

Vitamin C is the main treatment for dry mouth. If you do have this condition, besides the suckable tablets by your bed, take daily:

3 500 mg tablets Vitamin C.
2 Vitamin E with Selenium tablets.
2 Blackcurrant oil tablets.

Short sightedness (myopia) and long sightedness

These two complaints are generally caused by eyeball distortion, causing the lens to improperly focus light onto the retina. It does not mean a damaged retina.

Long sightedness is much rarer than short sightedness. Although the effects are similar, it should not be confused with common, old age sight which usually starts from about 45 yrs upward, and is caused by a loss of the lens' ability to change focus at close distances).

A two minute laser operation (cost $4000 per eye) can be successful in mild cases of short sightedness. In severe cases, laser surgery can cause scarring of the cornea and the success rate is seldom more than 25%. Rectifying glasses generally give relief to such conditions.

Some people have confirmed to me that just taking vitamins A, C, E, and Selenium has healed their short or long sight and they have abandoned their glasses.

Children with myopia

Short sighted children are almost always found to be lacking in essential eye nutrients. Asian children appear to be particularly susceptible, with current rates up to 85%. Native South American and Pacific Island children on the other hand have only about a 2% rate.

A study of the eye pressures of 11 year old children found that those with the higher pressures had a higher chance of developing myopia than those with lower pressures. This would seem to indicate that nutritional supplements may well be necessary for some children, especially those with higher eye pressures.

My advice to children and adults with myopia; take Eye Bright Plus, Lutein, Bilberry, anti-oxidants, Vitamin A, C, E, Omega 3 oils, and CoQ10.

Keep a safe distance away from your TV

A Japanese study, concerned over the increasing prevalence of myopia in children, concluded that stress and long hours of close viewing (reading, TV or computer) was harmful, and if the close viewing concerned TV or computer screens it was even more harmful.

The magnetic disturbances caused by cell phones are minuscule compared to force fields surrounding microwave ovens and TV's.

Dry inflamed gritty eyes and a dry mouth

Often this condition can also be a symptom of far more serious conditions, such as Sjogren's syndrome, Lupus or Hashimoto's Thyroiditis. They are auto-immune diseases, suspected to be of rheumatic origin and can often be present for many months, or even years before they are properly diagnosed.

They attack the glands that produce both tears and saliva. They also attack and destroy the thyroid gland, causing a condition called hypothyroidism, which causes many eye problems.

At that stage hormonal thyroid supplements should be used. Ask your doctor to check your thyroid.

Lupus

If you have Lupus or any other auto-immune disease, be aware that they can and do affect your eyes in various nasty ways. This can include blocked or swollen veins which lead to decreased vision, bleeding and sometimes blindness.

Also an eczema-like condition can appear around the eyelids, the muscles in the eye can become swollen and inflamed, as can tissues around the eye, and the eye may become temporarily paralysed.

Itching, burning, lack of lubrication (tears), and a sensitivity to light are all part of the curse of lupus.

Lupus of course affects many body parts, but I am only relating it to eyes. Lupus is a rheumatic disorder and there are hundreds of various symptoms it hides under. It takes a very smart ophthalmologist to identify it at first inspection.

Conjunctivitis can also become common.

I noticed in a paper on Colloidal Silver that it has been successfully used against Lupus. Re-read what action to take against other eye problems with Colloidal Silver (page 43) and follow the same instructions.

No tears

In a normal eye, a watery solution provides lubrication and to stop this watery lubrication from drying out too quickly, the lacrimal gland applies a coating of oil to the outside layer.

Auto-immune problems slow down this production of tears and oil, causing eyes to be dry, itchy, gritty and feel as if they are burning.

They also become very sensitive to light. On a windy day these symptoms may feel even worse.

I would take the same mineral, vitamin and herbal supplements as suggested for dealing with Macular Degeneration.

Less common eye troubles

Retinitis Pigmentosa (RP) This fairly rare eye trouble can often be misdiagnosed as Lupus, Sjogren's syndrome, Hashimoto's syndrome or Thyroiditis.

It is found that people with Retinitis Pigmentosa are more prone to develop those troubles. In fact these five problems are often similar and may be found together.

They are regarded as auto immune conditions. That means that the cells in the body fight one another.

When the eye becomes involved in such battles, it means inflamed or blocked veins or haemorrhages which can lead to decreased vision or blindness in some cases.

Orbital Myositis This eczema-like condition can occur around the eyelids and the muscles become inflamed or swollen, or even temporarily paralysed.

Sjogren's Syndrome This is often misdiagnosed. Like Lupus it is an auto-immune and rheumatic problem and some symptoms are similar to Lupus.

The dry eyes and mouth are caused by the destruction of glands which produce tears and saliva.

But just because you have dry eyes or mouth is not to say you have this complaint. As pointed out elsewhere, Aspartame can cause the same symptoms, as can possibly other medical drugs.

It is suspected stress and viruses are responsible in some way for Sjogren's syndrome.

Floaters or spots before eyes These are most often caused by anxiety and stress, but can sometimes be caused by a malfunctioning liver. Herbs which normalise liver function often heal this condition.

They can also be caused by leakage of blood into the macula, the small, sensitive central area of the retina.

Red, inflamed or sore eyes Sometimes it feels as if a piece of sand is in the eye.

Bilberry, Vitamins A, C and E, Selenium, Zinc, Perfect Eyes (or EW) and Beta Carotene effectively solve this disorder.

Some medical eyedrops can actually cause this problem, so you will have to decide which you prefer.

Tired eyes and/or drooping eyelids Again Perfect Eyes or Bilberry will solve the tired part and I suggest Vitamins A, C, E and Selenium may well help the other.

Diabetes

The second largest cause of all blindness in the USA is diabetes.

Some researchers now agree that Vanadium and Chromium are essential to prevent diabetes. My latest information is that Vanadium in the form of vanadyl sulphate should be taken after meals at a rate of 20-70 milligrams, depending on weight.

Vanadyl sulphate is available without prescription in America but I doubt if it has been heard of in New Zealand. It is also reputed to be a muscle builder and is used by some body builders for this purpose.

Chromium is also essential for the control of diabetes. In August 1957 the American Journal of Science stated that, *"Diabetes can be prevented and cured in animals by the use of vanadium and chromium.'*

Some 30 years later the University of British Colombia Medical School put out a paper on the successful treatment of diabetes in humans by the use of Vanadium and Chromium which appear to have similar roles in the body.

Other nutrients deficient in diabetics

Potassium, Magnesium, Vitamin B12, Omega 3 oils and Thiamine are almost always deficient in diabetics.

It has also been found that with some diabetics, about 5 mg of Vitamin B6 per day has allowed them to do away with insulin.

Cold pressed flax oil has been shown to be beneficial to diabetics. Besides being a good source of Omega 3, flax oil increases the body's response to insulin.

The New England Medical Journal states that Omega 3 oils are very effective in overcoming insulin resistance.

Diabetics or people with hypoglycaemia should also be aware that the drug Prednisone destroys insulin in the body.

A new treatment of diabetes – AEP

Because diabetes is the second largest cause of blindness in the western world, I believe sufferers should not bind themselves to outdated methods of treatment when a better remedy is available.

In Germany at Lake Silbersee in Hanover, there is a hospital based on alternative medicine called Paracelsus Hospital. It was founded by a Dr Hans Nieper over 40 years ago.

At that time, two research scientists suggested to him that two new mineral substances they had discovered may have a medical application.

These substances were Potassium and Magnesium with an electrical charge and combined with an amino acid transporter called arginates or AEP.

These two minerals were later licensed as a medicine by the German Health Authority under the name of Vitamin Mi for the treatment of Multiple Sclerosis.

AEP a major breakthrough

The good doctor began using these two minerals on his patients and this is what he writes regarding diabetes Type 2, after more than 30 years of observation.

"The application of Calcium arginates (AEP) and Magnesium arginates (AEP) belongs to the most positive experiences in my entire life. The blood sugar drops in a most spectacular way.

In one case the administration of Calcium and Magnesium Arginate, dropped the morning glucose reading from 300 down to 134 with no change in diet. I think we made a major breakthrough in the control of this most vicious disease."

He also states *"The kidneys are the organs most endangered by diabetes on a long term basis. It is a diabetics fate to frequently suffer kidney failure and be connected to a dialysis machine. We have observed in 24 years of administering Calcium AEP that diabetic retinopathy will practically not occur."*

Retina of eyes protected

"Having collaborated with several ophthalmologists in Germany and the USA we are now certain that this therapy is extremely effective in retaining the function of the retina. The kidneys are also protected in a manner unimaginable up to now.'

Circulatory health benefits of AEP

"During the last 30 years we have been able to observe that for patients taking Calcium and Magnesium AEP, the development of thrombosis, circulation problems, high blood pressure, and the progression of varicose veins is almost entirely eliminated."

Asthma and MS success with AEP

"Now we have almost no asthma patients left, especially none of younger or middle age."

"While formerly one third of all MS patients would die of lost nerve function, and one third of increased tendency to bone fractures, and the last one third, of kidney failure, only two patients out of 2,200 did this."

Dishwash detergent and diabetes Type 2

Dr Nieper believes that one of the causative factors of Diabetes Type 2 is contact with residual detergent on dishes. He suggests that only Citric Acid be used in dishwashers and for hand-washing dishes.

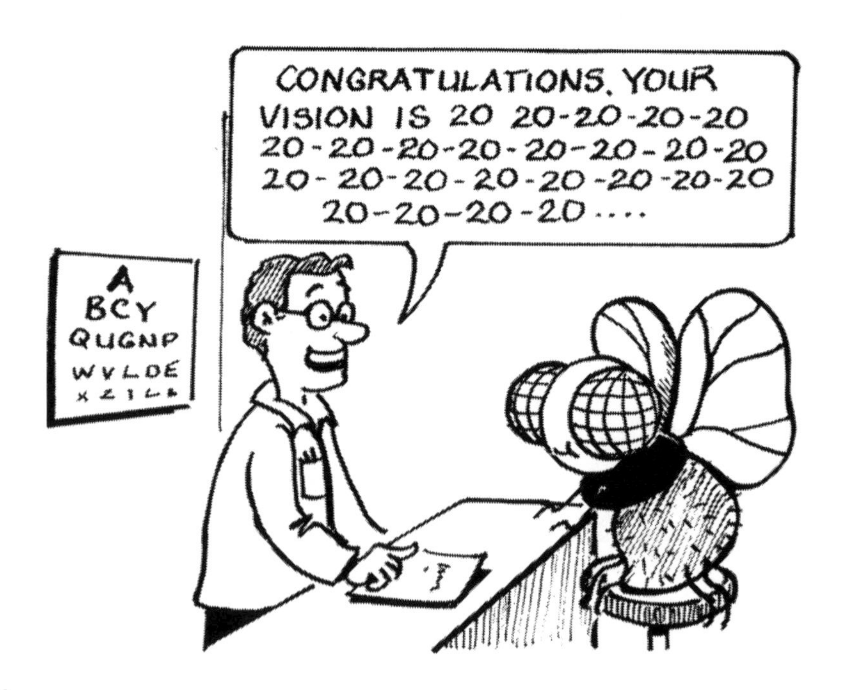

Minerals, vitamins and your health

The absolute certainty of life is that everyone must die. No matter what we eat or drink we cannot escape that appointment.

Nevertheless, research is showing that by ensuring that we have an adequate intake of the essentials for bodily health, we can considerably extend a useful and healthy lifespan.

Some of us now know that minerals, vitamins, enzymes, bioflavonoids and herbal extracts play an important part in healthy longevity. But as far as understanding what the maximum or minimum intakes necessary for good health are, we are only on the bare edges of such knowledge.

We now know that over 74 minerals have been isolated from human tissues, and so far over 60 of these have been found to interact with each other in various bodily functions. Many of these are only necessary in minute amounts, but without them the whole body cannot be perfectly attuned to excellent health.

Very little is done in medical school to train doctors on the advantages of mineral and vitamin treatments for deficiency complaints.

More research still needed

The supplements I suggest you take for eyes generally work for most people, but only time and research will tell if better results can be obtained from a higher or lower intake, and if other trace minerals are an advantage.

Some people say to me, *'Oh I don't need any of that stuff. I never eat anything but healthy foods!'*

But hang on, just what are healthy foods? Soil that has been constantly cropped for over 50 years contains virtually no Zinc and probably many other minerals are also seriously depleted. So no matter how many carrots, lettuces or cabbages you eat from such soils, there will be very little if any Zinc, Copper, Selenium, etc, in the vegetables grown on it.

Where do vitamins, amino acids and fatty acids come from?

They come from the foods we eat, or in some cases, our bodies manufacture them.

You cannot have healthy eyes without a healthy body, and the information in this book may help you understand what happens to your body when it is deficient in various minerals or vitamins.

Scientists have discovered that to operate at maximum efficiency, our bodies require the availability of some 60 basic minerals or elements (many in microscopic amounts only), some 16 vitamins and 12 amino acids.

Where do minerals come from?

Minerals in all cases come from the soil. Plants cannot manufacture minerals, nor can your body. If they are not in the soil they are not in the plants you eat.

Ten years of cropping depletes from soil most of the more common minerals in daily demand by our bodily mechanisms. How many commercial food growers or even organic home gardeners topdress their soil with minerals, apart from the three essentials, nitrogen, phosphorus and potassium (NPK) that all plants require?

And unfortunately, even if the soil has adequate minerals, many of these are lost through refining or processing of foods. Wheat loses about 70% of its mineral content when refined into white flour. It is discarded with the bran and germ and used mainly for animal feed.

As we age can we process minerals from our food as efficiently as the young?

No. Our absorption drops as we age. So the older we get, the more we need from our food.

It has been estimated that to obtain the minimum daily requirement of Zinc (provided it is in the soil) for a 70 year old, we would need to eat two and a half cups of split peas daily, (peas have the most Zinc of vegetables) or seven table-spoons of pumpkin seed.

So sometimes it is easier, and cheaper, to buy and

swallow a Zinc tablet than to consume all that food.

Even with young people, only 8 –12 % of some minerals in their food is absorbed by their bodies.

By the time they have reached 40 years of age the absorbtion has dropped to 3 – 5 %.

That is why it is of absolute prime importance for the elderly to ensure they obtain and use mineral-rich foods, water or tablets.

What is the best way for our bodies to acquire minerals?

By far the best way to acquire minerals is to drink them by way of colloidal mineral water, by drinking sea water if you have access to a clean supply, or by unrefined sea salt.

Sea water and unrefined salt contain traces of all 74 minerals.

However sea water and salt do not contain anywhere near enough of the major minerals we require. But it does help provide the ones we require in micro amounts.

What are colloidal minerals?

Colloidal minerals are minerals ground to almost atom size smallness and thus easily suspended in water.

Sea water is an example of minerals in a colloidal state. In their ultra-fine suspended state they are highly available to the human body.

Not only because they are so finely ground, but also because they contain a negative charge which appears to help their uptake by our bodies.

What are chelated minerals?

Chelated minerals are minerals that have been absorbed from the soil by plants, and combined with proteins and amino acids by the plant.

They are about 40% more absorbable by our bodies than those that have not been processed by plants.

Even though these minerals are extremely tiny, or atomised, they are not as tiny as those found in sea water.

A sea water health method

Take four litres of unpolluted sea water, well away from a river mouth or sewage outfall. Boil it gently for 20 minutes. Put it into a sterilised glass bottle (not a plastic container as it may eventually corrode it) and do not screw the top down hard.

Take one dessertspoon daily, either neat, or diluted in a glass of water, or put it in your porridge, stew or soup. Cooking cannot destroy minerals.

One dessertspoon of sea water contains one fifth of your bodies daily requirements of salt (sodium).

I have heard of one 91 year old man who has bathed his eyes twice daily with diluted sea water (besides taking it), and he claims his eyesight has shown great improvement over the 16 years he has used it. He started taking it at the age of 75.

Clean sea water is available to purchase in most Health Shops in America. Perhaps one day some entrepreneur in New Zealand will bottle it for sale.

Copper and Iron

Copper enables our bodies to absorb Iron. Iron is essential for our bodies to manufacture healthy blood. And healthy blood is essential for healthy eyes.

Illnesses associated with lack of Copper include ruptured aortic aneurism, cerebral aneurism, grey hair, skin wrinkles, varicose veins, sagging muscles and sagging breasts.

On the other hand, too high an intake in Copper can cause problems such as high blood pressure, anxiety, insomnia and hyperactivity, to name but a few.

Women on birth control pills are often found to have excess Copper levels. An adequate intake of Zinc, Selenium and Vitamin C generally deals with excess Copper.

Iodine

A shortage of iodine in your body will not allow it to process Vitamin A. This will in turn affect the thyroid hormones which control the rate our body can produce energy.

Before the introduction of iodised salt, goitre (an

enlargement of the thyroid gland to extract more Iodine from the blood) was prevalent in many countries. Goitre is again appearing in many countries as people use less iodised salt.

Besides goitre, a shortage of Iodine in young or old, results in a slowing down of bodily functions.

Iodine also helps control mucus. If you have a cough that seems to linger, test yourself for Iodine deficiency by trying this simple test. When you go to bed at night, paint about four square inches of your instep with tincture of Iodine. If the dark stain on your skin has gone by morning you are short of Iodine. Put on more Iodine. When your body does not need more Iodine the skin will remain stained, so don't put any more on for a few days. Painting your instep every few days is a simple and safe way to give your body Iodine as and when it needs it.

Why you need Calcium

A healthy body requires traces of all 60 minerals. Some of the really essential ones can give us big trouble if we don't supply them, Let's look at Calcium.

There are 147 deficiency illnesses associated with lack of Calcium. Among them, to name but a few are:

Bells Palsy **PMS**
Bone Spurs **Cramps**
Twitches **Osteoporosis**
Gall Stones **Kidney Stones**
Receding Gums (caused by osteoporosis of the jawbone)
Arthritis (85% of arthritis is caused by lack of Calcium)
High blood pressure **Insomnia**
Lower back pain (osteoporosis of the vertebrae).

Results of two Calcium experiments

An American experiment, lasting over 20 years and involving some 20,000 high blood pressure patients found that not taking salt in their diet made no difference whatsoever to their blood pressure.

A control group of some 5000 people had as much salt as they liked, but doubled their Calcium intake. This experiment was stopped after six weeks because by that time, 85% of these people's blood pressure had returned to normal.

Another experiment involving women with PMS. found that by doubling their Calcium intake, 85% of all emotional and medical symptoms disappeared

Kidney stones and gall stones

In March 1993, after a trial study of 4,500 people on Calcium intakes ranging from very low to high, the Harvard Medical School in Boston stated, *"A high calcium intake appears to limit the risk of developing kidney stones.'*

Very likely the same applies to gall stones. However once you have developed gall stones, taking Calcium will not remove them, but should prevent more developing.

On taking Calcium

Where Calcium is taken on its own, and it is often prescribed to women, there is a danger of calcification of the aorta of the heart if Magnesium is not also taken at the same time.

It is increasingly being recognised that Calcium and Magnesium work together, in a ratio of four parts Calcium to one part Magnesium.

Magnesium is now recognised as essential for eyes. It helps stop Calcium deposits forming in veins of the eyes which can be a serious problem.

Also when working or exercising hard enough to sweat, we need to supplement with Magnesium, as the more we sweat the more Magnesium we lose.

Some symptoms of Magnesium deficiency

Migraine headaches.
Eyelid spasms.
Leg cramps.
Asthma.
Back spasms.
Monthly female cramps.

A shortage of Magnesium also interferes with your body's uptake of iodine.

It is estimated that almost half of all medical problems arise from lack of exercise. It is here that Calcium seems to play a reverse role to chromium. Chromium in our body is only used and expelled when we exercise. The harder we exercise the more we need.

With Calcium, the less we exercise the more Calcium we lose, and the more we exercise the less we lose.

So daily exercise is a golden rule. At least half an hour a day.

What is osteoporosis?

Osteoporosis is a shrinkage of the bones due to an inadequate intake or uptake of Calcium.

The human body needs a minimum amount of Calcium daily, women more than men. Our bodies regard our bones as a Calcium bank. If we don't supply enough Calcium in our daily diet for 'essential services' then it withdraws Calcium from our bones. Calcium-deprived bones become thinner, porous, very brittle and actually shrink.

As a result we see people losing stature as they age. Some women can lose as much as 12 inches in height between the age of 50 and 70. And the slightest misadventure such as a fall can result in broken bones.

None of these troubles need happen if we take adequate Calcium and Magnesium daily.

Where can I get Omega 3?

The easiest way to obtain Omega 3 is to use plant oils or fish oils, but not just any plant oil.

Supermarket shelves are crowded with all sorts of plant oils, but despite all the promises on the labels, they are of no help to a healthy diet. This is because almost all of them have been heat-processed during extraction. Any heat over 100°C turns most good oils into bad oils.

Any health shop can supply you with a quality, cold pressed flax oil which is high in Omega 3.

Or you can buy ground Flax Seed (also known as ground Linseed). This dark brown flour has a 33% Flax Seed oil content, plus a lot of other goodness. You can use it in your baking or in your porridge. It is also very reasonably priced.

Stock thrive on it.

Have you been conned?

If you have been using margarine in preference to butter as a means to reduce your cholesterol, you have been conned. Margarines contain trans fats which can actually raise total cholesterol and LDL cholesterol more than butter.

Also any essential fatty acid oils found in man-made heat-processed fats such as margarine, are of little use to the body. They might look and taste the same as natural oils, but they are damaged beyond recognition during processing.

They are rather like a key that slides easily into a lock but fails to turn it.

About 80% of the cholesterol in our body is made by our own liver. Food only accounts for about 20%. Most of this comes from animal protein food such as meat.

For baking, the only oil I can suggest is cold pressed Flax Seed oil which is high in Omega 3. Cold pressed olive oil is okay, but contains little of essential fatty acids.

You must be discriminating in buying oils. Some manufacturers claim their oils are cold-pressed and they do not tell the truth. Some manufacturers also use solvents to remove the last vestige of oil from the processed waste, and in the process gather pesticides into the oil.

Any reliable manufacturer of cold pressed oil will pack it in a light-proof container.

So what is the best oil for cooking?

There is only one truly healthy cooking medium – WATER. So let's take a quick look at water.

It comprises about 75% of our body. In every breath we exhale we expel water, and most of us do not replenish our bodies with this life-giving element to the extent we should.

But don't binge on sugar and fats too often

The quickest way to hurry our aging is, according to research, to live our lives without discipline and eat too much and too often, especially sugary and fatty foods.

And it is essential to bear in mind that the worst possible fats you can eat are unnatural, man-made non-fats like margarine and hydrogenated oils.

The only oils of benefit to the human body are cold-pressed oils such as flax, coconut, palm, avocado and olive oil.

And it has also been conclusively proven that natural

animal fats in moderation are good for health.

But if you do partake of an enjoyable fatty meal, afterward flood your body with anti-oxidants, because oxidation of ourselves and excess sugar intakes are a nasty combination and hurry along all sorts of health problems. In fact, try to live without too many manufactured sugary foods.

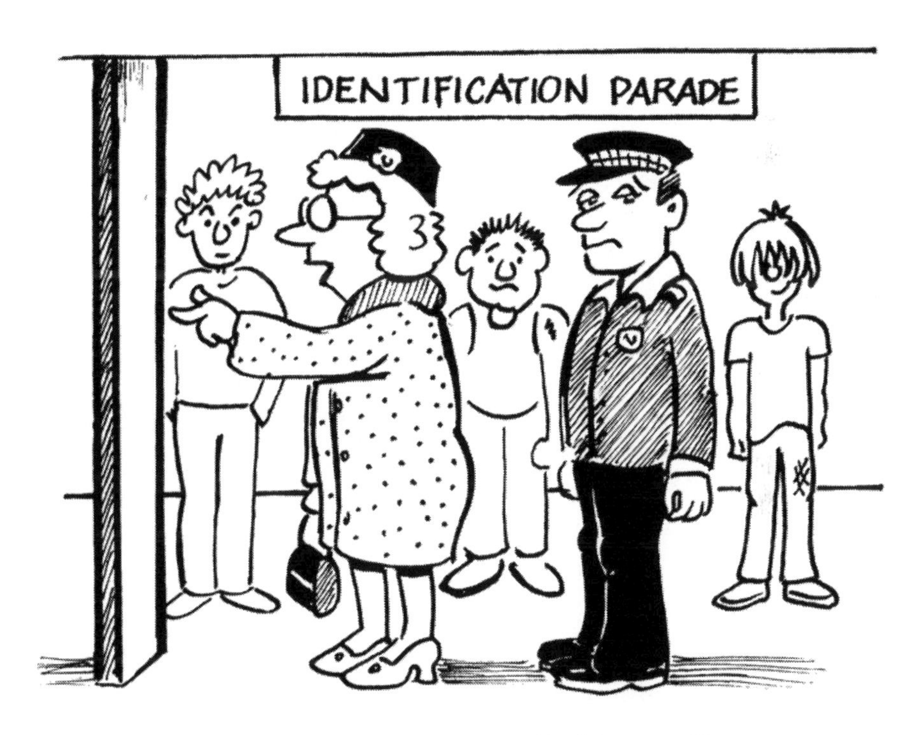

"That's him! The tall thin one!"

Looking at water

Over hundreds of years, medical advice has been to drink plenty of water. The modern recommendation is to drink eight ounces of water six to eight times a day.

How many people do this?

No. Drinking ten cups of tea or coffee, or four bottles of soft drink a day is not drinking water! These things are diuretics. They expel water from your body.

Dr Batmanghelidj's water cure for stomach ulcers and asthma?

Probably one of the most non-famous of doctors to graduate from St Mary's Medical School of London University in recent years is a Doctor F. Batmanghelidj.

I say non-famous, because he made a discovery that threw terror into the drug companies regarding two of their most profitable drugs – those for stomach ulcers and asthma.

In 1981 he discovered, in a trial of over 3000 patients with stomach ulcers, that in 95 out of every 100, their ulcers disappeared simply by drinking 8 to 10 eight ounce glasses of water a day. He stressed that it was important to drink a glass of water immediately before eating any meal.

And as a side effect of his research, with those same 3000 patients, he discovered that those who had asthma found it cleared up.

Black listed

The medical profession and the drug companies were aghast at the possibility of losing so many regular paying patients to something they could not patent or sell.

In fact the American Medical Association refused to even examine his research findings. So his name and research are on a very black list.

The good doctor presented his findings on asthma to the Interscience World Conference on Inflammation, Anti-rheumatics and Analgesics in 1989.

He claims ulcer pain will go within 20 minutes by

immediately drinking three glasses of water.

And asthma sufferers who would like to dispose of their nebuliser may well like to try this costless treatment. Try drinking 10 glasses of water a day.

If you can't manage this much, at least increase your water intake. But remember, no tea, coffee, soft drinks or anything containing caffeine or diuretics.

Blood pressure normalised and constipation cured

Many people on 10 glasses of water a day have found their blood pressure returned to normal.

Others with a history of decades of constipation returned to normal function.

I have always drunk water before, with, or after meals and at the age of 75 it has still never bothered me. Some say drinking water too close to meals dilutes enzymes necessary for good digestion. Well, you make your own decision about that.

Doctor Batmanghelidj has written a very intelligent book on his research entitled "Your Bodies Many Cries For Water." Buy a copy, or ask for it at your library.

More on water

Although we take it for granted, water is possibly the most important catalyst for removing fat. The most essential thing to do to keep fat away is to drink water. Water suppresses the appetite and helps our body burn fat.

Studies have shown that a decrease in water intake increases fat deposits, while an increase in water intake reduces them.

The reason for this is that our kidneys cannot function properly without adequate water. If they do not get it, some of their work is by-passed to the liver. An important task of our liver is to turn stored fat into energy.

If our liver is also doing some of our kidney's work, it cannot operate efficiently. As a result we have less energy, and more fat stays in our cells.

It seems a contradiction but – drinking more water is the best treatment for fluid retention

When the body does not get enough water, it perceives it as a threat to survival and sends out orders to hold every drop of fluid.

So water is stored outside the cells in extra cellular places. Thus swollen feet, legs and hands. (Poor heart valve function can also cause swollen legs.)

Diuretics are a temporary solution. They force out stored water all right, but along with it often go essential nutrients.

However the body perceives the diuretic as a threat and will replace the stored water at the first opportunity. Only when you give your body more water than it needs will you solve the problem of fluid retention.

Excess salt is sometimes a cause of fluid retention. The more salt you consume, the more water your body needs to process it. So the more salt you consume, the more water you need to drink.

Try to drink pure water

The less pollutants in your water the more efficiently it is set to work as a solvent, removing heavy metals, excess minerals, salts, etc. And the more quickly it can supply nutrients to our cells.

Our body does not regard tea, coffee, fruit juices, soft drinks, beer, milk or other liquids as water.

All our cells require water daily, just as much as they do oxygen and other nutrients. Water regulates all body functions and is essential for waste removal from our cells. Only with adequate water can our cells flush out wastes.

Water helps your muscles

Water helps sagging skin following weight loss. Shrinking cells are buoyed up by water, which pumps the skin and leaves it resilient and healthy.

Costless cures for some unpleasant ailments

The latter pages of this book offer some research findings that are almost costless cures for some unpleasant ailments.

Learn how to stay healthy

To start with, I cannot recommend too highly a book written by New Zealander, David Coory of Tauranga.

David's book is called "Stay Healthy by Supplying What's Lacking in Your Diet" and costs $25 couriered free.

It is written in a very easy to read style and deals with cholesterol, carbohydrates, alcohol, calories, fats, fibre, protein, sugars, minerals and vitamins. David points out what is necessary for good health.

He listed all the essential minerals and vitamins we need, what happens when we are short of them, and symptoms to watch for if we take too much of any mineral or vitamin.

He also lists the RDI (Recommended Daily Intake) of what medical researchers believe is all we need of this or that mineral and vitamin to stay healthy. He also lists the foods which contain a significant amount of each of these vitamins or minerals.

If you are of average intelligence you will have no trouble in understanding why you have suffered from various ailments over the years, but more importantly, you will understand what your body needs for good health and to avoid the pitfalls of the past.

On pages 140-141 of his book is listed over 70 ailments (including all eye disorders), which to quote, "*are being treated very successfully, without side effects by doctors who specialise in natural healing using mostly vitamin and mineral supplements. Often in high doses and skilled combinations and sometimes with herbs for heightened effect*".

David now has a website listing his book, my book and other NZ health books. It is www.zealandpublishing.co.nz.

Natural cure for gallstones

Here is how two women I know removed their gall stones painlessly within 24 hours by using this natural remedy.

Take two cups of lemon juice and two cups of olive oil. Shake them together.

Take a dessertspoon of the mixture every 15 minutes until you have taken the lot. Then lie on your right side.

They both passed their stones painlessly within six hours of taking the mixture.

One of the women, who was in severe pain before taking the mixture, stated that the pain continued for five hours, then stopped, and has never returned.

The other woman, who was told she had to wait three months for an operation, decided not to wait in pain that long. She passed 61 stones, two of them as big as marbles, and never felt any pain.

An experiment with hopeless arthritis patients

In September, 1993 the Harvard Medical School, who had been conducting experiments at their VA Hospital with arthritic patients who had shown no response to any other treatment, conducted this experiment with 29 people using ground-up chicken cartilage.

(A substitute product is available in grocery stores in the USA under the name of Knox Gelatine. Davis Gelatine in NZ is probably similar.)

They gave each patient two heaped teaspoons of ground chicken cartilage in one glass of pure orange juice, every day.

Within ten days all pain was gone. Within 30 days they could open a screw top pickle or jam jar, factory sealed. And in 90 days, all functions were normal.

I suspect there is a lot of Calcium in chicken cartilage or Gelatine and if I had arthritis I would certainly try this experiment.

Repetitive strain injury

Most of us have heard of people with a condition called RSI (Repetitive Strain Injury). A painful pins and needles feeling caused by compression of nerves in the wrists. The medical profession call it Carpal Tunnel syndrome and say the only cure is an operation.

Mineral and vitamin researchers tell us taking a proper balance of vitamins and minerals will usually see the problem totally disappear in most sufferers.

Fibrocystic Breast

A Canadian experiment in 1988 on a number of women with a painful condition called Fibrocystic Breast, showed that the symptoms would completely disappear if they took elemental iodine. When they stopped taking iodine the condition returned, showing that Fibrocystic Breasts are caused by iodine deficiency.

Obesity

There are people genetically disposed to not metabolise food as well as most. They have my sympathy.

But with most of our population, the problem of obesity is caused by wrong foods and over eating.

Wrong food and drink destroys health

Many people almost live on Kentucky Fried, McDonald's, fish and chips, pies, and drink nothing but beer, fizzy drinks, or tea and coffee.

They rarely drink water. They over-indulge in tobacco, alcohol, sugars and fatty foods. As a result they become grossly overweight and at a very early age develop all sorts of medical problems.

They then visit the doctor for a magic healing potion. It does not exist.

They will not take his advice about healthy eating, so what else can a doctor do except prescribe a few drugs which may keep them away from his surgery for a few months.

The fact is, that the only way to a healthy lifestyle is to learn the rules for a healthy, trouble-free body, and to abide by those rules. Well, most of the time anyway.

Aspartame (951)

Have you a nasty eye problem? – perhaps it's caused by Aspartame

What you might ask is Aspartame?

It is an artificial sweetener, which is deadly for the eyes of some who use it, often without knowing. 54% of Americans now consume it in their food or drink, mostly unaware of its dangers to health, especially their eyes.

Side effects of Aspartame

Here are some of the side effects of Aspartame:

Blindness.
Pain in the eyes.
Dizziness.
Macular degeneration.
Diabetic retinopathy.
Decreased vision.
Double vision.
Inexplicable retinal detachment and bleeding.
Irritated eyes.
Difficulty wearing contact lenses.
Convulsions.
Swollen infected eyelashes.
Memory loss.
Dry eyes.
Dry mouth.

These last two disorders can often be misdiagnosed as Sjogren Syndrome. Aspartame has an affinity for the saliva and tear glands, hence the dry eyes and mouth.

In 1986, the Community Nutrition Institute in Washington appealed to the FDA to ban Aspartame which they had formerly approved, because of links to blindness and eye problems in many people, but was turned down.

More recently, a report by Dr H.J. Roberts on Aspartame, after studying some 800 users with inexplicable eye problems, states that:

25% of users had suffered decreased vision.

8% of users suffered severe eye pain, dry eyes, dry mouth, leg cramps and joint pains.

Most of the symptoms were reversed over a period of one month when no more Aspartame was used.

A statement by Dr J. Bowen to the FDA in America states, *"Every known metabolite* (what remains after metabolism by our body) *of Aspartame is of marked questionable toxicity and patently unsafe for humans."*

50% of Aspartame is Phenylalanine (which converts to Formic Acid in the body or when warmed to over 30°C). Other components are Aspartic Acid and Methanol.

Methanol in our bodies converts to Formaldehyde (embalming fluid) in the retina. As little as 10 cc of Methanol taken internally can cause blindness and paralysis of the optic nerve.

In a quick survey of a New Zealand supermarket in Wairoa, I found Aspartame in low-calorie sweeteners, diet soft drinks and chewing gum. So if you value your eyes – be warned.

The food additive code number of Aspartame is 951. Watch for it.

Regard Aspartame as a tiny dose of nerve gas you deliver to your body each day

This story of Joyce Wilson of Stockbridge, Georgia, USA is told by her husband.

"My wife Joyce was a woman full of life, not overweight, but wanting to stay slim. When NutraSweet was approved by the FDA of America, she thought it was a diet product, not a drug."

"So she used sugar-free chewing gum, the low calorie sweeteners 'Equals' and 'Slimfast' and drank diet drinks."

"She gained 35 lbs (16 kilograms)."

"I saw her going down and tried to get her off it, but she said, 'It would not be on the market if it was not safe."

"She went to thirty-four doctors trying to find an answer, but the truth was concealed. With FDA approval she was consuming a deadly poison."

"One ophthalmologist saw the damage to the optic nerve and thought it was Macular Degeneration. No one knew that the Methanol (wood alcohol) in Aspartame converts to Formaldehyde in the retina of the eye."

"One day, Joyce, who was now blind, heard Shannon Roth, who had also been blinded in one eye by NutraSweet, explain her injuries."

"Joyce said, 'That's me,' and phoned Shannon and learned that NutraSweet is a deadly poison."

"Next, Joyce saw Dr Morgan Raiford, the renowned ophthalmologist who founded the Atlanta Eye Clinic. He was a specialist in Methanol toxicity, having treated moonshine victims during the era of American prohibition. He confirmed that Joyce was being blinded by NutraSweet."

"Joyce had been wrongly diagnosed as having Multiple Sclerosis (MS) because the doctors did not know that Methanol toxicity mimics MS as it destroys the nervous system. She suffered terrible headaches, hypertension and tachycardia, rapid heart beats; all Aspartame symptoms."

"She did everything she could to help other victims. She testified before a congressional committee and received an assurance from the FDA that they would not approve it for any other products without consulting her committee of Aspartame sufferers."

"Thirty six hours later the FDA approved it for other products. At that time it was only in 500 products. Today it is in 5000. Monsanto is the drug company that make Aspartame."

"Joyce died in 1991."

"Remember, Aspartame only has side effects in 1% of users, but who knows what sort of genetic effects could be passed on to the next generation by the constant use of this nasty product, especially to the unborn if their mothers use it during pregnancy."

Other nasty drugs

There are thousands of medical drugs on the market, and a great many of them have nasty side effects. Here are some of the worst:

Ritalin This drug, widely prescribed to keep over-active children quiet, can suppress weight and height, and cause seizures, insomnia, anorexia, nervousness and dependence.

Prozac (also sold as **Sarafem**) A drug used to treat major depression and obsessive-compulsive disorders. 10% of people using it are at risk of violent behaviour or suicide. Other side effects are anorexia and insomnia. More recent information links it to side effects throughout the whole body, including sexual dysfunction.

Septrin An antibiotic sulpha drug. Can kill blood and liver cells. Has been known to cause Stevens-Johnson Syndrome (SJS), a severe skin rash which can often be fatal.

Lariam. An anti-malaria drug, but there are severe side effects for some users: hallucinations, seizures and nasty mood swings.

Prednisone (also sold as **Predisolone** and **Prednisolone**) A steroid, and like any steroid used for any purpose except for a short time, it can have nasty side effects, including dementia, osteoporosis and retarded growth.

Sodium Valproate An anti-epilepsy drug that has many side effects, including liver failure in some people.

Piroxicam (also sold as **Feldene**) Anti-inflammatory non-steroid drug. Can cause stomach perforations or bleeding, hair loss, depression and over 100 other side effects.

Nifedipine Calcium blocker. Dangerous to diabetics. Increases risk of suicide, depression, bleeding of stomach, cancer, heart attack.

Cancer questions

What is cancer?

Cancer is a body condition where cells begin to chaotically multiply, sometimes very slowly, sometimes very rapidly.

How does orthodox medicine treat cancer?

Three ways – 1. Surgery.
2. Burning (radiation).
3. Poisoning (chemotherapy).

How successful are these methods?

Some succeed, some don't. A USA report in 1987 said that the overall age-adjusted death rate for cancer had hardly changed in recent years. It went on to say, *"For the majority of cancer patients we examined, the actual improvements have been small and overstated."*

Which treatment has the worst failure rate?

Chemotherapy. Consider these words written by Ulrich Abel, a German cancer researcher. Ulrich wrote to some 300 Cancer Research centres around the world, seeking any encouraging results from chemotherapy.

As a conclusion to his findings he published this in a German science magazine a few years ago. *"Chemotherapy is a scientific wasteland. But is so entrenched in the minds of both doctors and patients as an effective treatment, that neither group is willing to stop, even though there is no evidence it prolongs life."*

What about surgery?

It helps some. But in 20% – 60% of cases, depending where the cancer is, some cancer cells are left behind, allowing the malignancy to regrow.

How about radiation?

Can be useful to slow down cancers, but rarely cures.
Can weaken the immune system.

How effective are alternative treatments?

When we consider that patients that take alternative treatments have first tried orthodox doctors who have been unable to help them. Also that their bodies are riddled with cancer and they have only weeks to live, alternative treatments are quite successful.

When successes occur in these patients given up for dead, the medical profession cries, “Spontaneous healing!”

But remember this, spontaneous healings occur at the rate of about one in 10,000. Alternative treatments run miles ahead of that rate, even though they start with a nearly dead patient.

Does orthodox medicine research alternative treatments?

Almost never. Ralph Moss, an American cancer research journalist, states this of alternative treatments, *"44% of treatments are condemned out of hand, and most others are condemned from hearsay, not research or trials."*

What is the focus of alternative treatment?

It is based on stimulating the body's own natural defence mechanisms to fight the disease.

This is done by way of herbs, minerals, vitamins, proteins, amino acids and raw foods.

In the case of Dr Hans Nieper, it also involves taking orally, substances that help repair genetic information destroyed by cancer cells.

In another case, destroying cancer cells by very low voltage radio waves over certain frequencies.

Are most of the people who practice alternative treatments dumb fools?

No, the bulk are disillusioned doctors, many with very high qualifications, or scientists, (some of them Nobel prize winners) who found they were fighting a losing battle with the dogmatism of the American Medical Association to obtain recognition of improved treatments.

Are the people who patronise alternative treatments of low intelligence? No, most are very well educated.

Where can I learn more about alternative cancer treatments?

There is an excellent book I read recently called "How To Fight Cancer and Win" by Professor William L. Fischer.

He is not a medical doctor but a scientist. His book explains cancer research and treatment, plus the use of essential fatty acids (omega fats) and food diets to kill cancer. It is a 342 page book and the price is about $50.

How effective is chemotherapy?

For some strange reason, Western medical associations, appear to be possessed by a mystical obsession that the only cures for medical problems, especially cancer, will come from the pharmaceutical giants.

Woe betide any person or doctor who successfully treats and cures a person another doctor has pronounced 'terminal'.

Consider what Dr Hardin Jones of Berkeley, California University had to say in 1975 after a 20 year study of chemotherapy. *'Patients are as well off, or better off, untreated'.*

Chemotherapy is a huge money spinner. Drug companies in America currently sell doctors $8,500,000,000 worth of chemotherapy drugs each year.

Yet there are hundreds of doctors throughout America who have successfully treated cancer with alternative medicine. When discovered, they have been forced out of practice by the AMA.

Can the body repair DNA cell damage?

This quote is from an article published in the German magazine Raum und Zeit. I quote:

"Even though large specialised hospitals have not acknowledged the fact, it is nevertheless true, that extraordinary expensive chemotherapy and radiology are without a doubt a failure."

"The internationally recognised Oncologist, Dr Hans Nieper from Hanover, Germany reports in this article – 'A Promising Therapeutic Possibility in Conquering Cancer', namely the application of active substances from plants (and insects) for

the repair of genetic (DNA) information which got lost in cancer cells."

(Editors Note. The two substances are Dionaea, made from the Venus fly trap plant and Irrododial, made from ants, and are now widely available.)

Breast cancer self-healed 30 years ago by DNA repair

Regarding the genetic repair of the body's DNA, consider this 30 year old German report:

"In 1973, in the Silbersee Hospital in Hanover, Germany, a so called spontaneous healing of advanced breast cancer was witnessed. The healing process in itself was very dramatic.

With the help of monies given by the Volkswagen Automobile Company, the cancer patient was given extensive tests. The results obtained seemed to show that the cause of the drastic disappearance of wide spread cancer metastasis throughout the bones of the patient, had its foundation in the ability of the body to repair a derailed genetic system in the cancer cells and not with the usual immune system response, as with people responding to bacterial or viral infection."

Natural remedies soon priced off the shelves?

Freedom to buy natural health remedies in NZ may be coming to an end

Sadly, the days when we can prescribe to our own health with the use of minerals, vitamins and herbal remedies may be coming to an end. Drug companies and most doctors have declared open war on herbal and supplement companies and the health products they sell.

Already in some countries, the supplements we can purchase over the counter in New Zealand or America have now by political decree been banished from the shelves.

Natural remedies have become so popular world-wide that the drug barons have taken action. They are buying out, or pricing out the opposition.

The power of the multinational cartels.

Because of their immense wealth and power, the multinationals are generally the biggest sponsors of medical research in almost all the medical universities in the Western World. They thus control in which direction medical research moves.

They make certain that any university endeavouring to research minerals or herbal treatments runs short of sponsors very rapidly.

Consider this, would any drug baron tell you how to live a long and healthy life, during the course of which you would be so healthy you would never use any of his drugs?

Buying out the opposition

The world-wide vitamin manufacturing company 'Quest' is now owned by Boehringer, one of the largest pharmaceutical companies in the world.

Other big drug manufacturers are buying out herbal and vitamin companies.

With the immense wealth of the pharmaceutical companies behind them, these natural product companies can, by heavy advertising, completely swamp the smaller companies and force them out of business. Or they can sell similar products at a much lower price, until the opposition is bankrupted. The way is then open to raise their prices so high as to force us all back into seeking relief from their high profit, unnatural, manufactured drugs.

Why would giant pharmaceutical companies want to banish natural remedies that have been used successfully for thousands of years? There is only one answer, greed for gain.

They know that natural remedies contain thousands of healing substances, and unlike their present drugs, they have almost no side effects. Well, why don't they research and test herbal remedy extracts and market them?

No reason, except that they would then want to patent that product and raise the price 30,000 times above cost. (Yes some drugs are marked up that much!) And who will pay them that sort of money, if people can walk into a health shop and buy a tablet that does the same job for 30 or 40 cents?

Just my imagination running riot you think? Well consider this; Dr Charles Moertal discovered a sheep deworming drug called Levamisole, which he tested on 1300 human patients. Although the drug had side effects, it reduced colon cancer by 41% and the death rate from that illness by 33%.

A farmer could purchase enough Levamisole treatment for 30 sheep for $7. When sold from a pharmacy for humans, the cost to treat just one person was $200 per month.

Canada moves to abolish natural remedies

Hand in glove with the pharmaceutical giants, Canada has commenced to do what Germany and the Scandinavian countries have already nearly completed; they have drawn up savage penalties to outlaw health shops and herbalists.

They are forcing every manufacturer of a dietary supplement, claiming any health benefit, to apply for a DIN (Drug Identification Number) at a cost of $720 for each named supplement, and a yearly renewal of $500.

Already they have banned the following natural remedies from being imported or sold in Canada.

L-Arginine (Amino Acid) Cardiovascular support.
L-Carnitine (Amino Acid) Combats heart disease.
Chaparral (Herb) Anti-oxidant and anti-inflammatory.
Chromium Picolinate (Mineral) Useful for diabetics.
Cramp Bark (Herb) Relieves menstrual cramps.
EPA (Fish Oil Extract) Improves circulation.
Eyebright (Herb) Essential to relieve many eye problems.
Glucomannan (Vegetable fibre) For treating obesity.
Germanium (Mineral) Improves immunity.
Goldenseal (Herb) Treats cold and flu symptoms.
Gotu Cola (Herb) Improves memory, promotes relaxation.
Hawthorne Berries Heart tonic.
Horsetail (Herb) Source of silica.
Melatonin (Sleep Hormone) For insomnia and a jet lag.
Octasanol (Wheat Extract) Counteracts fatigue.
dl-Phenylalanine (Amino Acid) Natural pain killer.
St Johns Wort (Herb) Mild tranquilliser.
L-Tyrosine (Amino Acid) Natural anti-depressant.
Yellow Dock Root (Herb) Astringent.

Pau d'arco and **Uno de Gato (Cat's Claw)** Two South American vines that are powerful anti-viral and anti-fungal agents. Excellent for reducing side-effects of chemotherapy. They have also proved effective in reducing many cancers, including brain tumours. The Indians of Peru have used them for centuries as all-purpose healers.

(I strongly recommend you read the book written by Kenneth Jones entitled *"Cats Claw, Healing Vine of Peru."* The information may save your life.)

DHEA (Natural Hormone) As we age, our levels of DHEA decrease year by year. The lower the levels, the more prone we are to disabilities of old age. People who supplement with DHEA have been found to maintain far better health. It is freely available from all health shops in America, but was banned from importation into New Zealand in 1997.

New Zealand and Australian governments are now lining up to follow Canada to clamp unnecessary controls on most vitamins, minerals and herbs, especially those that give far more effective results than pharmaceutical drugs.

All the health products mentioned above have now been banned in Canada as a first step. The penalty for importing or being found in possession of any of them makes you liable to a term of imprisonment between 18 months to 10 years.

Far more than the few health products listed above have now been banned throughout Germany and Scandinavia.

Be alert to any sly moves in NZ

Well, readers, I could say much more, but please be alert to any sly moves by our politicians (accompanied by much propaganda on the dangers of self treatment) to ban or make manufacturers pay exorbitant registration fees for natural remedies.

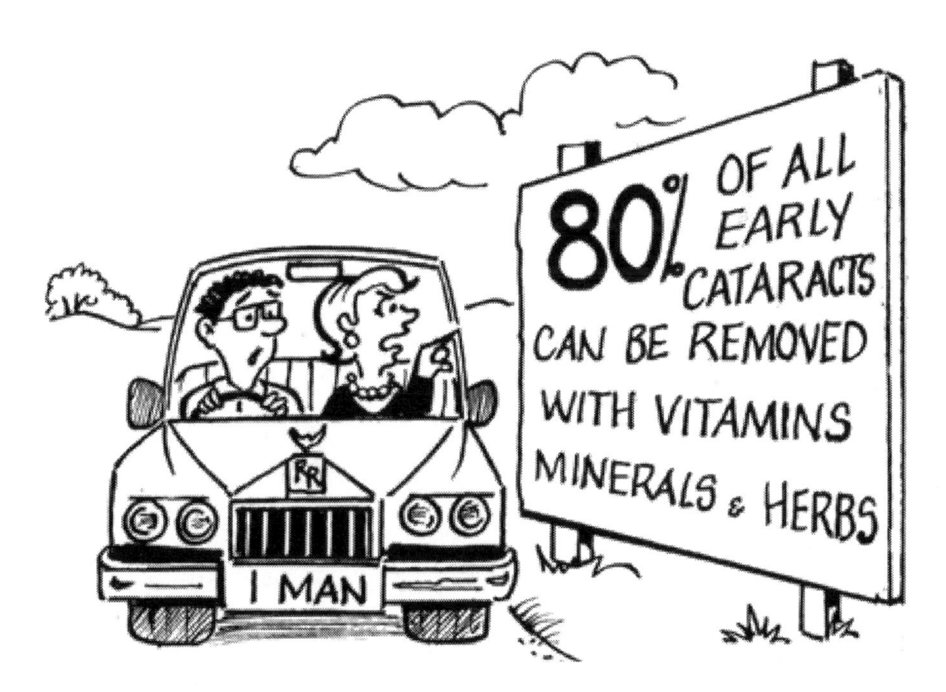

"If this keeps up George, you'll be back to driving a Toyota."

How many die in New Zealand from drug side effects?

Last year we heard a great chorus of complaints from the Health Department because a woman in New Zealand died from an overdose of herbal tea.

How many women have been killed in New Zealand by wrongly prescribed or administered pharmaceutical drugs?

The fact is, that any 20 herbal remedies mixed together and taken daily are thousands of times safer than any five pharmaceutical drugs taken simultaneously.

Hospitals' and doctors' mistakes with drugs are buried deep in New Zealand. Only by vigorous ferreting by reporters, do mistakes receive any glare of publicity.

This is due to our antiquated libel laws, which state that it is unlawful to publish any article about a company or person, even if perfectly true, if that statement damages their reputation. So in New Zealand, one can be sued for telling the truth.

Fortunately in America, the truth is more respected. We read of an article dated 13 January, 1993 published by Ralph Nader (of Consumer's Rights fame), in which he states 300,000 PEOPLE ARE KILLED IN AMERICAN HOSPITALS EACH YEAR AS A RESULT OF MEDICAL NEGLIGENCE. That's over three times the annual road toll in the USA.

All of these deaths are caused by either doctors prescribing the wrong drugs, the side effects of a drug, adverse results from mixing of drugs, or medical staff misreading a prescription.

Until Ralph Nader 'blew the gaffe' few people knew that the killings were occurring because the medical death certificate would state, *'Iatrogenic causes'* (a complication of medical therapy).

We do not have a Ralph Nader in New Zealand. I wonder how many death certificates written in this country list *'Iatrogenic causes'*.

The blackout in medical schools about Colloidal Silver

I am astounded by the almost total lack of knowledge among the medical profession about the deadly efficiency of Colloidal Silver against a whole spectrum of illnesses caused by fungi, bacteria and viruses.

Ask almost any nurse, doctor, pharmacist or vet about Colloidal Silver. Most of them have never heard of it. So the suppression starts right at the top.

Can you think of a reason why? There is a very simple reason – money.

Consider this – if a bottle of Colloidal Silver could cure colds, shingles, whooping cough, sore throats, athletes foot, and all of the hundreds of illnesses caused by fungi, viruses or bacteria within a few hours, or a day or two, how many people would be visiting doctors?

The pharmacist would have a savage drop in income too. Hardly anyone would be coming in with prescriptions.

And don't forget the pharmaceutical drug industry. If hospitals could make their own Colloidal Silver on the premises so cheaply, they could swab the floors with it, to whom would the drug barons sell their unneeded products?

Daring to speak out

I have received some letters from opticians and doctors thanking me for the information in the first edition of this book and congratulating me for *"daring to speak out"*.

Their words have emboldened me, so I tell the medical profession to shake off the shackles of their union and form a 'breakaway union' that will insist that they be allowed to teach and practice whatever heals their patients.

At present, any doctor who advocates a healing procedure that does not have the approval of his 'union bosses' can be struck off the medical register.

So almost all unwillingly keep silent.

Setting the inflexible rules

The rules for 'medical industry' are always set by the top brass in the drug and medicine industry who want nothing to do with cures if cure means a drastic loss of income.

They decide what young doctors will learn, and what they will not learn in their university and hospital training.

And it is what is not taught in supposed universities of knowledge that is costing taxpayers in the so-called civilised world billions of dollars in totally wasteful and unnecessary expenditure in health budgets.

What motivates doctors?

A survey of medical students in an American Medical School in early 1980 discovered that 84% of them were not training to be doctors because they wanted to help heal people, but because they considered it a highly paid job.

One can only wonder, after years of example by our political leaders to *'look after number one'* if any different result would be found among New Zealand medical students.

A money sucking scandal

What needs to be done to stop this money sucking of the public purse scandal? Not to mention the years of unnecessary pain and suffering by people with shingles and similar ailments?

In my opinion, nothing less than a commission of enquiry into all these aspects of modern medicine and some very valid reasons why such a totally harmless substance as Colloidal Silver should not be used for the benefit of humanity.

Outdated methods

There are dozens of areas that I and other people who practise alternative health can point out where orthodox medicine causes governments and their citizens to pay out vast sums of money on outdated methods of treating ailments. Shingles, chicken pox, conjunctivitis, etc. In fact any of the 600 plus complaints caused by fungi, viruses or bacteria.

Well I have said my piece, and maybe I have been outspoken. But all is not as it could be in the medical industry.

It is now up to you.

I am sure that what I have put before you in this book, if acted upon, will have a beneficial effect on your eyes. Also on your general health in other body areas.

It is now up to you.

If you are seeking one pill that will cure your eye problems, you will find no answer in this book. Good health in today's world demands that you must personally learn to recognise your body's deficiencies and take action to supply what is lacking.

Where the facts in this book came from

Apart from relating what happened to myself regarding glaucoma, the information regarding eyes and health in this book has been gleaned from the journals of Ophthalmology, the Townsend letters to doctors, journals of the AMA, The Lancet and University Research publications.

I hope by using the information within these pages, you can improve, or at least hold your vision for more years than otherwise have been possible.

I thank all those people who provided me with helpful information to make this knowledge available.

Printed in Great Britain
by Amazon